Dr Vasundhra Atre

HEARTBEAT

How to prevent a heart attack

With Best Wishes

Vasundhra

PopulaR
prakashan
www.popularprakashan.com

Published by
Harsha Bhatkal for
POPULAR PRAKASHAN PVT. LTD.
301, Mahalaxmi Chambers
22, Bhulabhai Desai Road
Mumbai - 400 026

© 2015 Vasundhra Atre
First Published 2015

(4422)
ISBN: 978-81-7991-863-0

General Disclaimer
The medical information in this book is only for the purpose of general education and not intended to be a substitute for actual medical diagnosis and advice. While the presented information is based on reliable reputed sources and full care is taken to avoid any errors, the dynamic nature of medical science and concepts makes it imperative that readers should always check the accuracy of facts with their doctor.

The opinions in this book are solely those of the author. Popular Prakashan Pvt. Ltd. assumes no responsibility for the content.

Design: Anjali Sawant
Typesetting: Satyawan Rane

PRINTED IN INDIA
by Saurabh Printers (P) Ltd.
Plot No. 67 A-68, Ecotech, Ext. I
Kasna, Greater Noida-201306 (U.P)

In loving memory of my father,
who encouraged me to dream
and gave me the belief that
'Everything is possible'.

Contents

Foreword

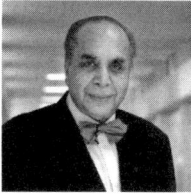

Coronary artery disease is a killer worldwide. The focus of management of coronary artery disease has over the years shifted from just early diagnosis, treatment and crisis management to trying to understand risk factors and managing them better.

Coronary artery disease is progressive. The heart does not protest unless serious blocks have already developed or the heart is being pushed beyond its limits. An understanding of the problem, will help one understand the importance of regular check-ups, the need to address any complaints at the earliest and motivate one to make the lifestyle changes necessary for a healthy heart.

In her twenty-year journey as a cardiovascular thoracic anesthesiologist, Dr Vasundhra Atre has conducted over 10,000 cardiac related surgeries and in the process has developed an excellent understanding of coronary artery disease.

In this book, she has exhaustively addressed all the questions that are normally asked by patients and their families about coronary artery disease. The information succulently addresses all aspects of the disease process, diagnosis, age and gender differences, medical and surgical interventional management and the preventive aspects.

Dr Atre has written an excellent guide to understanding coronary artery disease in a simple and comprehensive manner, which will be really useful to the patient and their families.

— Dr B K Goyal
FRCP (EDIN), FRCP (LON), FAMS, D.Sc (HON), FACC, FSCAI
Director, Cardiology,
Bombay Hospital and Medical Research Centre
Former Recipient of Padma Shri,
Padma Bhushan and Padma Vibhushan

Foreword

Heart ailments are a leading cause of death in India. With our genetic make up, the Indian Diaspora across the world is susceptible to Diabetes Mellitus and accompanying heart diseases. The burden of our changing lifestyle and environmental pollution is going to make India the diabetes capital of the world. With this grim scenario in mind, it behooves us to learn about the disease and take preventive steps to delay and alleviate such ailments.

It is not possible to change our genetic make up but we can definitely make important changes in our lifestyle to prevent a heart disease. As a cardiac anesthesiologist, present at numerous heart operations, Dr Vasundhra Atre has minutely observed the details of the operative findings and has made useful suggestions through this insightful book.

Heartbeat is a common man's guide on what to do if one suffers from a heart attack. It also out lines the appropriate measures and resuscitation efforts that can be carried out. I trust this book will become popular and help patients suffering from heart diseases to take proper precautionary measures as well as the general public to help them live a comfortable and productive life.

— Dr D S Saksena
MBBS, FACS, FACC, DABS, DABTS, FIACS AND D.Sc (HON) CSK
Hon. Professor and Head, Department of Thoracic and Cardiac Surgery,
Bombay Hospital and Medical Research Centre
Hon. Surgeon Commodore in Armed Forces Medical Services
The Commander of the Order of the Star and Key of the India Ocean

Preface

There is hardly a family where atleast one person is not suffering from a heart related ailment. The first time it is diagnosed is traumatic for both the person suffering and the family. Suddenly words like ECG, ST changes, coronary arteries, coronary blockages, ECHO, angiography among others need to be dealt with.

My journey of over 10,000 cardiac surgeries has given me a keen insight into the problem that is Coronary Artery Disease (CAD) or simply put the blocks that occur in the blood vessels of the heart that cause heart attacks.

The heart is an amazing organ; it starts beating in the womb and ticks till the end. It has a tremendous adapting capability and only starts protesting when it can't be pushed any more.

CAD develops over time. Often, conditions like diabetes, hypertension, thyroid related problems etc, which predispose one to the development of coronary blocks co-exist. If a patient comes to the operating table for a coronary bypass surgery or the cardiac catheterization laboratory for an angioplasty, he is there because of the cardiac risk factors that he carries. Unless, he understands those risk factors and tries to negate them in future, the disease is likely to progress or recur.

While working in the cardiac theatre, I often wondered at the triggers that caused the final insult resulting in the heart attack. Since the blocks do not develop overnight, why is it that the patient seems fine one moment and is experiencing a heart attack the next?

This led me to analyse the risk factors in my patients. In addition to the lack of proper diet, exercise, and associated conditions, like diabetes and hypertension, stress kept emerging as an immediate trigger. The factors that account for stress vary from person to person—be it a set back in business, death in the family, meeting deadlines, or the neighbour's television being played at full volume every night!

We live in an era of easy access to information. In the earlier years the questions that were asked pertained more to the disease process and what was being done about it. Today, there is an attempt to understand 'why it happened', 'my options', and 'what can I do to prevent it from happening again?'. As medical consultants, we explain the 'condition' to the patient and expect them to comprehend everything in that one consult. My experience as a caregiver made me realise that even as a medical specialist I had many unanswered questions when it came to taking care of my dear ones in times of illness.

This triggered a desire to write on medical issues in an easy to understand manner. I have been contributing to the wellness section of a leading newspaper in India since 2002 and have contributed over 1000 web pages for a medical encyclopaedia.

This book is an attempt to offer comprehensive and complete information on all aspects of coronary artery disease in a simple manner.

Heartbeat, essentially attempts to answer all questions regarding coronary artery disease that my patients and their families have put to me. Right from the structure of the heart, to the disease process, risk factors that can cause coronary artery disease, what to do when you suspect that a heart attack is occurring, the preventive routine tests and their interpretation, tests that could likely be advised if coronary artery disease is suspected, their significance and interpretation.

As soon as someone mentions the fact that he or she has a heart ailment; the advice and different modalities of treatment suggested are unending. All coronary artery disease cases do not need surgery and all coronary artery disease cases cannot be managed by medicine or alternative treatments either. An understanding of the different options available and the possible reason behind the options being offered helps decision-making, ensuring that the best treatment is offered. This book is an effort towards explaining the possible rationale behind the available modalities.

Topics like heart disease in women, in children, in those with thyroid issues are also touched upon.

An insight is afforded into the various new 'cures' that are being explored and the ones that offer hope, in the future, for those suffering from coronary artery disease.

Using technology to keep risk factors in check and also for an early diagnosis could prevent progression of the disease and also limit the damage to the heart muscle. Ways to understand your body type, making the right choices and importantly sections on possibly preventing and reversing heart disease are also included in the book.

After all, prevention is better than cure.

— **Dr Vasundhra Atre**
MD, MPhil HHSM (BITS Pilani)

Acknowledgements

Writing acknowledgements is a pleasurable task. It reminds me of all the help and support I received in making this book a reality.

I would like to thank my family, my senior doctor colleagues and friends for their unlimited support and continuing encouragement.

A special thanks to my patients and their families, who asked relevant questions which, motivated me to write this book.

I am grateful to my publisher Popular Prakashan for publishing this book. I would also like to thank Swapna Shinde, Gauri Rane Shetty, Armaity Motafram and Anjali Sawant for their invaluable inputs and their faith in me.

Chapter 1

Coronary Artery Disease: The Facts

The heart is an organ that beats tirelessly from the womb to the end. Continuous, uninterrupted blood flow to the heart muscle ensures that it gets the oxygen and nutrients that it needs to keep beating.

When we talk about Coronary Artery Disease (CAD) or Coronary Heart Disease (CHD), it means that there are blockages in the blood vessels that supply the heart. Any interruption to the blood supply of the heart muscle causes it to protest resulting in a heart attack.

All of us know someone who either has a heart problem or has suffered from a heart attack.

The following are some of the myths and facts about CAD:

The Myths

- Men are more likely to develop coronary artery disease as compared to women.
- A heart attack is the problem of the guy next door, not mine.
- Stress alone cannot cause coronary artery disease.
- A normal ECG means I do not have a heart problem.
- Once I have been diagnosed as a heart patient, my life becomes restricted.
- At thirty I am too young to have a heart problem.
- Once I have heart disease I cannot do anything about it.

The Facts

Once considered a disease of the wealthy countries, today 80% of the 17 million deaths caused by heart disease occur in low and middle-income countries.

Before we go further, let us take a moment to review the following facts:

- Cardiovascular diseases are the leading causes of death worldwide.

- Coronary heart disease (leading to a heart attack) and cerebrovascular disease (leading to a stroke) are the two most common types of cardiovascular disease.

- Low and middle-income countries carry more than 80% of the global burden of cardiovascular disease. By 2020, deaths from cardiovascular diseases will rise to four million per year in China and almost five million in India.

- Eighty per cent of the cases of premature heart disease, stroke and diabetes can be prevented.

- Smoking, high blood cholesterol and high blood pressure are the three important preventable causes of these diseases. The risks of these diseases have been shown to decrease by stopping smoking, reducing cholesterol and reducing blood pressure.

(Sources: Preventing Chronic Diseases: A Vital Investment, WHO Global Report, Geneva, Switzerland, 2005; Global Health Risks: Mortality and Burden of Disease Attributable to Selected Major Risks, WHO, Geneva, Switzerland, 2009. The Global Burden of Disease: 2004 update WHO, Geneva, Switzerland, 2008. Surveillance of Mortality and Cardiovascular Disease (CVD) Related Morbidity in Industrial Settings, WHO Country Office for India, Geneva, Switzerland.)

The Indian Scenario

- The Indian Census in 2011 estimated the population of India to be 1,210 million, spread over an area of 32,87,268 sq. km.

- It is predicted that almost 2.6 million Indians will die due to Coronary Heart Disease (CHD) by the year 2020; i.e., 54.1% of all deaths in India will be due to CVD.

- CHD in Indians occurs prematurely, at least 10 to 20 years earlier than in their counterparts in developed countries.

- Demographic and health transitions, gene-environmental interactions and early life influences of foetal malnutrition are the likely causes of increased CVD in India.

The Cardiac Facts

Every second, a person suffers from chest pain or a heart attack in some part of the world. According to the *American Heart Association Update 2011:* "On the basis of 2007 mortality rate data, more than 2200 Americans die of CVD each day, an average of 1 death every 39 seconds."

Headlines and news articles such as these have become common place:

Thirties are the new fifties for heart disease
Times Of India, Sept 25, 2009

The Saffolalife Study 2009, covering 8,469 people, found that 49.1% Indians were at high risk for developing heart diseases

By Malathy Iyer |TNN

. . . *Cardiologist Dr Manjeet Juneja, who consults at Wockhardt Hospital, Mulund, says heart disease is occurring 15 years too early for most people because of 'preventable causes'. He recalls a 23-year-old brought to the hospital from Nashik. "The boy was tense about admission to an MBA course and smoked a cigarette 30 minutes before collapsing," says Dr Juneja. He was managed with medicines alone.*

The irony — Dr Manjeet Juneja from Wockhardt Hospital, 39 years of age - fit and agile died of sudden cardiac arrest.

Burnout?
SAP India MD Ranjan Das dies of heart attack
ET Bureau, Oct 22, 2009

MUMBAI/BANGALORE: *Ranjan Das, managing director of SAP India, died of a heart attack on Wednesday. He had been at the helm of the Indian operations of the top enterprise software maker since 2007.*

. . . *In the past few years, heart attacks have claimed a number of high profile victims in the IT industry starting with the former chairman of Nasscom, Dewang Mehta. His death, which came just as the software industry was gaining prominence, occurred quietly and unexpectedly in a Sydney hotel a few months before he turned 40.*

Shortly afterwards Nasscom lost another of its senior leaders, Sunil Mehta, who was 41, to a heart attack. Another well-known name in the software industry, Arun Kumar, who was chairman of Flextronics, also passed away after a heart attack . . .

Ranjan Das was just 42-years-old.

We read these articles, go 'tch, tch', 'how sad', 'so young' and go about our business as usual. In our minds heart related issues are always the problem of the person next door. Health is taken for granted. We work hard and party harder, late nights and erratic routines have become a way of life. We subject the body to all sorts of abuses and still expect that it will not complain.

When it comes to health related issues we are all ostriches. We do not like labels such as 'hypertensive', 'diabetic' or 'heart problems' to be attached to us. So if we do not have regular check-ups, the problems do not get identified and of course, that means we are healthy!

Articles such as these should actually make us sit up and ask ourselves whether we or someone close to us could be the next victim.

Chapter 2

Understanding Coronary Artery Disease

I. Blood Flow to the Heart

"There is an average of one death every 39 seconds due to a heart problem . . . one heart attack every second somewhere in the world . . ."

The size of a fist, the heart is located beneath the breastbone in the chest cavity, towards the left between the lungs. Structurally it can be compared to a muscular house with four serially connected rooms – two upper chambers called the atria and two lower chambers called the ventricles. The two upper chambers are separated from each other, as are the two lower chambers, by walls called septa i.e., the atrial septum and the ventricular septum respectively. The heart valves, which can be compared to doors are located between the serially connected chambers and only open in the forward direction.

The heart has an inherent electrical supply that flows in a synchronized manner through the four chambers. Continuing with our analogy, the coronary circulation, i.e., the blood supply to the heart can be compared with the plumbing system in a house. It runs on the surface of the heart supplying it with blood, oxygen and nutrients needed to keep it working.

Functionally, the heart is a pump, made up of muscle. Its inherent electrical activity causes synchronized contractions, which push the blood forward into the circulatory system through the arteries to the body tissues and organs, providing them with oxygen and nourishment and finally taking the blood back to the heart through the veins (Fig. 1).

The heart in a normal adult pumps around five litres of blood. The blood is continuously circulated; a cycle takes around 60 seconds. Blood from all parts of the body is brought to the right upper chamber, from where it is pumped to the right lower chamber and then to the lungs where it is oxygenated. It then flows back to the left upper chamber and subsequently to the left lower chamber from where it is forced into the circulatory system.

The heart develops in the fifth week of pregnancy *in utero* and actually starts beating when the embryo is just six weeks old. From then on it continues to beat, throughout one's life at a rate of about a hundred times a minute, which is about 100,000 times a day, or 36.5 million times a year!

An amazing organ, the heart only complains if something goes wrong with either its electrical system, its plumbing system or if the walls or valves get damaged.

The Coronary Circulation

To enable the heart to continue its incessant beating uninterruptedly, it needs a good blood supply. The coronary arteries that supply blood to the heart muscle ensure adequate oxygen and nutrients for its activity. The coronary arteries are the first arteries to branch off from the aorta - the large artery that takes blood to the body from the left ventricle.

Normally, there are two main coronary arteries. The right coronary artery mainly supplies the muscle of the right ventricle, whereas the left main artery almost immediately divides into two branches - the left anterior descending artery and the left circumflex artery, which supply blood to the rest of the heart muscle (Fig. 2).

The main coronary arteries then divide into many smaller branches, which supply all the heart muscle. Any narrowing or blockages of these coronary arteries is referred to as coronary artery disease. The severity of the problem depends upon which artery is blocked and to what extent.

Coronary Artery Disease

Coronary Artery Disease (CAD), as the name implies suggests damage to the coronary arteries. The arteries become narrow and hardened, due to various factors including the natural ageing process.

The coronary arteries supply the heart muscle with oxygen and nutrition so that it can carry out its functions. Build up of fatty deposits i.e., plaque, on the inner wall of the coronary arteries causes them to become narrow and thick (Fig. 3). This built up of *plaque*, known as atherosclerosis, happens slowly and progressively.

While the exact cause as to why atherosclerosis occurs remain unclear, it is suggested that it begins because the innermost layer of the artery (the endothelium) is damaged. The possible causes of damage to the arterial wall include high blood pressure, elevated levels of cholesterol and triglycerides in the blood, and cigarette smoke.

Due to the damage, the walls of the inner vessel become rough, encouraging the deposit of cholesterol, fats, calcium and other substances from the blood. These substances in turn may stimulate the cells of the artery walls to produce other substances. These accumulating cells and the surrounding material cause the innermost layer of the artery to thicken. If the wall thickens sufficiently, the diameter of the artery reduces and less blood flows, thus decreasing the supply of oxygen and nutrition to the heart.

Plaques may be *soft* or *hard*. Hard plaques consist mostly of calcium and scar tissue, while soft plaques contain more of the cholesterol material. Soft plaques are considered more serious as they have the potential to rupture, get into the blood stream and cause sudden blocks further down in the artery.

As the plaques increase in size the coronary arteries get narrower (Fig. 4). This results in less blood flowing through them. As the plaque continues to accumulate, blood flow to the heart muscle progressively decreases and may even be cut off completely. The result is that the heart muscle is unable to carry out its functions properly, as it does not get enough oxygen and nutrition. The heart now complains, this is perceived as '*angina*', i.e., chest pain or discomfort experienced when the heart muscle does not get enough blood, oxygen and nutrition. It may feel as if there is pressure, a heavy weight or a squeezing pain in the chest. The pain can also occur in the arms, shoulders, back, neck or jaw.

When the blood supply or most of the blood supply to a certain part of the heart muscle is suddenly cut off, it results in a '*heart attack*'. If the blood supply is not restored in time the heart muscle can suffer permanent damage.

Disruption of the blood flow to the heart can affect the electrical circuitry of the heart. This can result in an irregular heartbeat or rhythm disturbances (arrhythmias), in which the synchronized pumping action of the heart is affected. Unless promptly and adequately treated some arrhythmias can be serious and life threatening.

Over time, coronary artery disease can weaken the heart muscle leading to heart failure. The heart is now unable to pump blood effectively to the rest of the body. This can lead to secondary problems as other organs, like the kidneys, receive less blood flow and may develop problems.

Atherosclerosis and build up of plaque are also responsible for the increased occurrence of strokes and disease of the peripheral arteries.

So, how do the coronary arteries get damaged?

II. The Risk Factors

The dictionary defines risk as anything involving exposure to danger.

A risk factor is exposure to something that increases your chances of getting a disease. There are several factors that increase the risk of developing Coronary Artery Disease (CAD). The greater the number of risk factors one is exposed to, the greater are the chances of developing CAD.

Some of these risk factors are within our control; these are known as modifiable risk factors. Others, which are beyond our control, are known as non-modifiable risk factors.

It appears that the risks are determined while a child is still in the womb. David Barker, a scientist in Southampton, England found that babies with a lower birth weight had a higher risk of dying from heart disease later on in life.

What We Cannot Change

There are number of factors that are beyond our control such as:

Age: As one grows older, the risk of developing coronary artery disease increases. Based on data from the Framingham trial, nearly 50% of males and 30% of females over the age of 40 will develop coronary artery disease. Other factors that are probably contributing to coronary artery disease being diagnosed almost a decade earlier among the Indian population are the increasing number of young people suffering from diabetes and hypertension, and the smaller calibre of vessels in the Indian population.

Gender: Men have always been considered to be at a higher risk for developing coronary artery disease. However, today, women are also facing higher risks.

Heredity and race: We cannot decide the family we are born into. Those with a family history of coronary artery disease inherit a tendency to develop the disease. African Americans have a higher risk of heart disease than Caucasians. The risk of heart disease is also higher among Mexican Americans, American Indians, native Hawaiians and some Asian Americans.

The study *Coronary heart disease in Indians: Implications of the INTERHEART study* authored by Vamadevan S. Ajay and Dorairaj Prabhakaran published in the Indian J Med Res. 2010 November; 132(5): 561–566; doi: 10.4103/0971-5916.73396 summarized the key results of the South Asian component of the *INTERHEART study*. It states:

- Deaths due to acute myocardial infarction (AMI) in South Asians occur at 5-10 years earlier than the western population.

- South Asian men encountering AMI were 5.6 years younger than women.

- The higher risk for AMI in South Asians in their younger age is largely determined by the higher levels of risk factors and the nine conventional risk factors (abnormal lipids, smoking, hypertension, diabetes, abdominal obesity, psychosocial factors, consumption of fruits and vegetables, alcohol and regular physical activity) collectively explain 86% of the AMI risk in south Asians.

- Abnormal Apo-B/ApoA-1 ratio and smoking are the most important risk factors.

- Low education level is associated with increased risk of AMI worldwide.

- Protective lifestyle factors such as leisure time physical activity and regular intake of fruits and vegetables are markedly lower among South Asians than western population, while harmful risk factors such as elevated ApoB/Apo A-1 ratio are higher in south Asians.
- South Asians have significantly higher population attributable risk associated with waist-hip ratio.
- Higher level of risk factors in both cases and controls under the age of 60.
- Regular alcohol consumption is not protective for AMI in South Asians (OR=1.06; 95% CI, 0.85–1.20).

What We Can Change

Modifiable risk factors, given below, can be modified, treated or controlled.

High blood pressure: The arteries are subjected to extra stress when the blood pressure is high. It also increases the workload of the heart.

High blood cholesterol: The risk of coronary artery disease increases with rising levels of blood cholesterol.

Smoking: Smokers face two to four times higher risk of developing coronary artery disease as compared to non-smokers.

Physical inactivity: An inactive lifestyle is a risk factor for CAD.

Obesity: Overweight or obese persons are more likely to develop heart disease and stroke even if they have no other risk factors.

Diabetes: Diabetes increases the risk of heart disease.

Stress: An individual's response to stress may be a contributing factor.

Alcohol: Consuming too much alcohol can raise blood pressure, cause heart failure and lead to a stroke.

High Blood Pressure and the Heart

Healthy arteries are strong, elastic and flexible. Their smooth inner lining allows the blood to flow freely, adequately supplying the vital organs and tissues with nutrients and oxygen. When a person suffers from high blood pressure, the increased pressure at which the blood flows through the arteries damages the inner lining of the arteries. This triggers the process of atherosclerosis which causes the arteries to narrow and harden; leading to narrowing of the coronary arteries and deceased blood supply to the heart muscle.

If a person suffers from high pressure, the heart has to work harder to pump blood to the rest of the body. This results in thickening of the walls of the left lower chamber of the heart (the left ventricle). The walls begin to stiffen or thicken (left ventricular hypertrophy). As a result of these changes the ability of the ventricle to pump blood forward is limited. The result is an increased risk of heart attack, heart failure and even sudden cardiac death.

The strain of high blood pressure on the heart causes weakening of the heart muscle and reduces its efficiency. Any added damage due to a heart attack aggravates the problem and the heart simply tires and fails.

Diabetes and the Heart

Diabetes is unfortunately only associated with a high blood sugar level. However there is much more to it than that. Diabetes is a metabolic disorder, which damages the nerves and blood vessels resulting in damage to almost all organs of the body.

Persons suffering from diabetes are not only twice as likely to suffer a heart attack as compared to non-diabetics, but they also have a tendency to develop heart disease or suffer a stroke at an earlier age. What is even more dangerous is that a diabetic person may suffer a 'silent' heart attack with no symptoms, since diabetes can damage the nerves resulting in no pain being experienced during the attack. In addition, heart attacks in diabetic patients tend to be more serious and are more likely to result in death.

Diabetics can suffer from microangiopathy, i.e., damage to the small blood vessels and capillaries and macroangiopathy, which damages the inner lining of the arterial wall, again accelerating the process of thickening and hardening of the vessel walls. All these factors contribute to coronary artery disease and its consequences.

Smoking and the Heart

Persons who smoke are two to four times more likely to get heart disease and two to three times more likely to die from heart disease.

Tobacco smoke contains nicotine, carbon monoxide and other dangerous substances.

- These cause damage to the arterial inner lining promoting atherosclerosis and triggering coronary artery disease.
- Additionally, smoking increases the stickiness of certain cells in the blood causing them to clump together and form blood clots. These sticky platelets can block the coronary arteries resulting in a heart attack.
- It can also cause the arteries to go into spasm, narrowing the lumen of the coronary arteries, reducing blood flow to the heart muscle and causing a heart attack.
- It can trigger irregular heartbeats.
- Smoking tends to reduce the level of 'good cholesterol' increasing the chances of developing plaques.
- It also reduces the amount of oxygen carried by the red cells, effectively decreasing the oxygen being delivered to the body tissue.

Smoking thus results in changes that cause damage to the arterial walls, cause the formation of plaque, narrow the blood vessels and reduce the oxygen carrying capacity of the blood – leading to an increased occurrence of coronary artery disease and other diseases.

Obesity and Heart Disease

Obesity simply describes the condition of anyone significantly above his or her ideal healthy weight. It is the result of consuming more calories than are burnt by daily, physical activities. Obesity is the result of too much fat being deposited in the body. These deposits of fat, especially around the waist can lead to:

- An increase in both the blood cholesterol and triglyceride levels.
- A decrease in the levels of 'good' cholesterol HDL, which in turn increases the risk of heart disease and stroke.
- An increase in blood pressure levels.

- Diabetes, which compounds the already existing other risk factors and further increases the risk of a heart attack.

Stress and the Heart

Today, it is not uncommon to hear even children and young people saying that they are stressed. Stress seems to be a natural fallout of modern day living.

What is this stress? Stress is the body's way of responding to any kind of demand. The body has an inbuilt survival instinct. When faced by a perceived threat the body responds with a 'fight-or-flight' response - the stress response. The body is flooded with adrenaline and cortisol. As a result the heart beats faster, the pulse rate increases, the muscles receive more blood, fats are released into the blood for energy, the muscles get tense, the breathing rate increases, the blood clotting ability increases – in other words the body is preparing to run or stay and fight.

The body responds in the same way, whether you are standing in front of a speeding truck or have had a bad day in the office. The body does not know the difference. It is just under stress.

Not all stress is 'bad'. Two types of stress are described, positive stress or 'eustress' and negative stress or 'distress'.

- Positive stress keeps 'the adrenaline pumping'. It is eustress that compels us to follow our dreams and realize aspirations. It is what keeps us going.

- Negative stress or distress, drains a person and leads to 'burn out'. Distress is what one experiences during a tragic event in one's life such as the death of a loved one, loss of a job, or even a bad interview.

How an individual handles stress decides the effect it has both physically and mentally. Consider the following:

- Do you think of a disagreement with a colleague as a part of working together or as a conflict?

- If you have a deadline do you use it as a way of getting the job done or think that it is your boss's way of troubling you?

- A colleague cracks a joke at your expense. How do you respond? Do you laugh at yourself or get offended?

It is up to you to decide whether you want to use stress to your advantage or allow it to affect your health.

Constant stress can affect you mentally, physically and emotionally, resulting in:

- Your heart beating faster, and working harder.
- Speeding up the blood flow, causing a rise in blood pressure.
- The release of fatty acids into the blood for energy causing the blood cholesterol and triglyceride levels to rise.
- The release of cortisol causing fat to be deposited in the abdominal region; the harbinger of health problems.

Alcohol and the Heart

Drinking too much alcohol can cause an increase in the fat levels – the triglycerides - in the blood. High blood pressure, heart failure and obesity due to an increase in calorie intake as also diabetes are the possible problems that can occur as a result. It can also lead to cardiomyopathy, a condition, in which the heart becomes enlarged, thick and rigid. The heart muscle is unable to function effectively and fails over time. Consumption of too much alcohol can also result in cardiac arrhythmias and sudden cardiac death.

Physical Inactivity and the Heart

Physical inactivity is said to double the risk of heart disease. A sedentary lifestyle translates into fewer calories being burnt. The result is, gain in weight, which in turn increases the risk of developing high blood pressure and type 2 diabetes, contributing to ageing of the heart. *The heart is a muscle; it needs to be exercised regularly to keep it fit.*

Know Your Fats

Every time high blood pressure, diabetes, obesity and heart disease are talked about there is always a mention of lipids, cholesterol and triglycerides; these are the reason why the arteries are damaged.

Lipids are fats, which are found in the body, however not all fats are bad for the body. Fats provide an essential fatty acid called linoleic acid, which is important for growth, healthy skin and metabolism. Fats also help absorption of fat-soluble vitamins (A, D, E and K) and of course, add flavour to food, making it tastier and more satisfying.

Cholesterol is a waxy substance found in foods from animal sources, namely, eggs, meats, and whole-fat dairy products (including milk, cheese and ice cream). Cholesterol is also manufacture by the body. The liver produces about 1,000 milligrams of cholesterol daily. Fruits, vegetables and grain do not contain cholesterol.

Cholesterol is needed to build the cell walls, produce Vitamin D as well as some hormones and even produce the bile salts, which help us to digest the fats that we eat. However, too much cholesterol in the body can lead to serious problems like heart disease. Many factors can contribute to high cholesterol, but the good news is there are things you can do to control them.

Cholesterol by itself cannot travel through the bloodstream. Certain proteins act as transporters to move it to different parts of the body. Together the protein and the cholesterol form a lipoprotein. High-Density Lipoproteins (HDL), the 'good cholesterol' and Low-Density Lipoproteins (LDL), the 'bad cholesterol', are the two most important ones. They are said to be good and bad because they have different effects on the body.

LDL cholesterol is more likely to block the blood vessels, interrupting free flow of blood through the body. HDL cholesterol actually helps to remove the cholesterol from the blood vessels and transport it back to the liver, where it can be treated and removed from the body.

The dictum is to keep the HDL cholesterol levels high, since it is good for you and the LDL cholesterol levels low since it is bad for you. Remember 'H' for high and 'L' for low.

Monitoring your cholesterol levels is important. When the level of LDL cholesterol increases, the cholesterol gets deposited on the walls of the blood vessels and forms plaques. This causes narrowing and hardening of the blood vessels, leading to atherosclerosis, which is the forerunner to heart attacks and strokes. It can also damage other organs like the kidneys.

Certain factors are associated with higher levels of bad cholesterol. These include:

- Being overweight.
- A family history of cholesterol or heart disease.
- A diet high in cholesterol, saturated fats, and trans fats.
- Ageing.
- Physical inactivity tends to decrease HDL levels.

The American Heart Association recommends that cholesterol intake should be less than 300 milligrams a day, total fat intake should be 30% or less of the total calories consumed, saturated fat should be 10% or less of the total daily calories, and trans fats should be less than 1% of the total calories consumed.

Other Possible Causes

It is not uncommon to come across someone with coronary artery disease who says, "But I do not have any of the risk factors. I am 30, there is no family history, I have no 'bad habits', I exercise off and on and am not overweight. How did it happen to me?"

A lot of research is being carried out to study other possible factors. They are as follows:

- **Sleep apnoea** is a disorder in which there are cycles when one stops breathing and then starts breathing again, whilst sleeping. When a person stops breathing the blood oxygen level drops suddenly which causes a rise in blood pressure and puts a strain on the cardiovascular system, probably predisposing to coronary artery disease. Anybody with a history of snoring should get checked for possible sleep apnoea.
- **C-reactive protein** is a normal protein. It is measured by a blood test and indicates inflammation and is used as a marker in certain diseases. High levels of C-Reactive Protein (CRP) may be a risk factor for heart disease. It is suggested that as the coronary arteries narrow, the CRP in the blood increases.
- **Homocysteine** is a non-protein amino acid. A product of the metabolism of the amino acid methionine, it is recycled like

the other amino acids. The body needs sufficient amounts of dietary Vitamin B12 and folate for the recycling. When there are inadequate levels of B12 and folate in the diet, the recycling process becomes faulty, resulting in an increase in the blood homocysteine levels. Studies suggest that abnormal levels of homocysteine in the blood may damage the lining of blood vessels, making the veins and arteries more susceptible to blockage or blood clots. This, in turn, may increase the risk of coronary artery disease and stroke.

- **Fibrinogen** is a protein in the blood that plays an important role in blood clotting. Increased fibrinogen levels cause platelets (blood cells responsible for clotting) to clump together. This can result in clots forming in the arteries causing a heart attack or a stroke. Fibrinogen can also be an indicator of the inflammation that accompanies atherosclerosis.

- **Lipoprotein(a)** forms when a low-density lipoprotein particle attaches to a specific protein. It can disrupt the ability of the body to dissolve clots. High levels of LP(a) may be associated with an increased risk of cardiovascular disease, especially coronary artery disease and heart attack.

Whatever the trigger, be it high blood pressure, diabetes or smoking, the basic damage occurs to the inner lining of the arterial walls, triggering build up of plaque with its resultant problems.

Having understood the possible risk factors for coronary artery disease, let us now see how to recognise a heart problem.

III. The Signs and Symptoms of Coronary Artery Disease, Heart Attack, Arrhythmias and Heart Failure

It is extremely important not to neglect any signs of health problems. A high index of suspicion is needed to diagnose a heart problem and get it treated in time.

Symptoms of Coronary Artery Disease

Angina or angina pectoris comes from Latin and literally means, 'squeezing of the chest'; it is the most common symptom of coronary artery disease. The hardening and narrowing of the coronary arteries, decreases the blood flow to the heart muscle, results in a mismatch between the supply and demand of oxygen to the heart muscle causing the heart muscle to protest.

This protest maybe experienced as a feeling of squeezing, pain, heaviness or discomfort in the chest that typically lasts from one to 15 minutes. The pain or discomfort may also be felt in the arms, jaw, neck, shoulders, throat or back. Angina is more often than not mistaken for indigestion.

Three attack patterns of angina are described as:

- **Stable (or chronic) angina** when the heart is made to work harder than usual, e.g., when you exercise. There is a regular pattern and this is predictable over time. The symptoms are typically relieved by rest or taking medication.
- **Unstable angina** on the other hand, has no regular pattern. It can occur even at rest, is less common and more serious. Rest or medicine does not relieve it. It can herald an impending heart attack within hours or weeks.
- **Variant (Prinzmetal's) angina** and **microvascular (smallest vessels) angina** are rare. These can occur at rest even when there is no underlying coronary artery disease. It is the result of *abnormal narrowing or spasm* of blood vessels causing decreased blood flow to the heart muscle. Medicines can relieve the angina.

Other symptoms of coronary artery disease include:

- A faster heartbeat.
- Shortness of breath.
- Weakness or a feeling of dizziness.
- Nausea.
- Clammy hands, sweating.
- Palpitations or what some patients describe as '*ghabrahat*' in Hindi which literally means feeling of uneasiness, irregular heartbeats, or a 'flip-flop' feeling in the chest.

Symptoms of a Heart Attack

The possible symptoms of a heart attack are similar to those for angina and include:

- A feeling of discomfort, heaviness, pressure or pain in the chest, arm, or below the breastbone.

- The discomfort may radiate to the arms, back, throat or jaw.
- There may be a choking sensation, feeling of fullness, indigestion or heartburn.
- Nausea, vomiting, sweating or dizziness.
- There may also be shortness of breath, and a feeling of tiredness and anxiety.
- The heartbeats maybe perceived to be very fast or irregular.

The symptoms during a heart attack typically last for half an hour or longer with neither rest nor oral medication giving relief. A mild feeling of discomfort can rapidly progress to severe pain. Some people may experience a silent heart attack, which means they have no symptoms at all. This is especially true in the case of diabetic patients.

Symptoms of Arrhythmias

When the electrical system of the heart is affected, abnormal heart rhythms (arrhythmias) occur. The rhythm may be regular or irregular, extremely fast or slow in nature, and is perceived as:

- A feeling of skipped heart beats, some kind of fluttering sensation or simply flip-flops in the chest.
- Pounding in the chest.
- A feeling of light headedness or dizziness.
- Shortness of breath.
- A feeling of weakness, or just tiredness.
- Fainting attacks.
- Discomfort in the chest.

Due to the disturbance in the rate and rhythm at which the heart is beating, the heartbeat (contraction of the pump) becomes ineffective. The resultant forward flow of blood to the organs and tissues is compromised resulting in the symptoms.

Symptoms of Heart Failure

If the heart muscle is pushed beyond a point, over a period of time it begins to give up and ultimately fails. Blood tends to stagnate both in the lungs and the peripheral tissues since the heart is unable to manage the circulation effectively. This results in the symptoms of heart failure which include:

- Shortness of breath during activity and even at rest especially when trying to lie flat.
- There may be productive cough with a white sputum.
- Swelling especially around the ankles, in the legs and abdomen
- Rapid weight gain.
- A feeling of dizziness.
- Excessive tiredness and weakness.
- Very fast or irregular heartbeats.
- There may be associated palpitations, chest pains or nausea.

It is very important not to neglect any discomfort or unusual symptoms. The best thing is to have regular medical check-ups. This will ensure that any abnormal values are picked up early and treated before any symptoms develop. Getting the right tests done at the right time is important.

Chapter 3

Evaluating Coronary Artery Disease

I. Take the Tests

"All that is wrong cannot be righted - be sure the wrongs are rightly sighted."

— Francis D. Moore

Most of us become health conscious after the damage is done. The reason for this is probably that so much is written and talked about coronary heart disease that everyone knows something, but is not familiar with all the details.

Getting the right tests done at the right time is extremely important. This is especially important for those who have a family history for any of the risk factors. They need to be more careful. Regular check-ups help identify the problem area/s early, allow timely lifestyle modification or treatment thus preventing the occurrence of heart damage. In fact a lot of health issues are identified during regular health check-ups.

One of the most frequently asked questions is, "At what age should I start worrying about heart health?" The present recommendations suggest that some basic screening should start early in life to identify risk factors, given below.

Basic Screening

Blood pressure: Blood pressure should be checked at least once every two years after the age of 20. If you have pre-hypertension or high blood pressure, your doctor may recommend more frequent screenings, periodic visits to his/her office and perhaps regular blood pressure monitoring at home as well.

It is not uncommon to have high blood pressure without any symptoms.

Cholesterol screening: A fasting lipoprotein profile (to measure total cholesterol, HDL, LDL and triglycerides) is recommended for all adults aged 20 and above, every five years. Depending on your risk factors for heart disease, your doctor may recommend more frequent testing.

Testing for diabetes: If you have a normal risk for diabetes you should start screening after the age of forty five. Persons who are 45 years and older are at risk for type 2 diabetes, and should have their blood sugar measured every year. Also, if you have high blood pressure or high cholesterol, it is important to be tested for diabetes, since diabetes significantly increases your already higher risk of suffering a heart attack.

Children who have been diagnosed as having type 1 diabetes early in life, and who may already be taking insulin must undergo regular check-ups and tests even before the age of 20.

Adults with a Suspected or Known Heart Problem

Adults who are suspected of having, or are known to have, a heart problem will require regular heart check-ups.

A cardiologist will carry out a primary clinical evaluation. Depending on any other existing risk factors and associated problems further consultations with an ophthalmologist, an endocrinologist/diabetologist or other specialists may be required and various investigations may be advised, which include:

Clinical Pathology
- Complete haemogram and blood group
- Urine: Routine and microscopic examination
- Urine: Microalbumin

Biochemistry Tests
- Blood glucose
- Lipid profile
- Apolipoprotein A[1], B
- Blood urea nitrogen (BUN)

- LP(a)
- Serum creatinine
- Serum uric acid
- Liver function tests
- Homocysteine
- hs-CRP
- Glycosylated Hb
- Thyroid profile

Plain Radiology
- Chest X-Ray (PA view)

Lung Function Tests

Cardiac Evaluation
- ECG
- Treadmill and other stress tests
- Echocardiography

Depending on what the above tests reveal further specific tests maybe suggested.

By now you are probably thinking: "So many tests! Why do I need to undergo so many tests? What are they going to tell me?"

Let us consider the tests one by one and understand what they mean and what they tell us.

Clinical Pathology

Clinical pathology aims to diagnose a disease by testing blood and other bodily fluids, tissues in the laboratory. It is a microscopic evaluation of individual cells.

- **Haemogram or Complete Blood Count (CBC) and Blood Group**

    CBC is used as a broad screening test to check for such disorders as low haemoglobin levels (anaemia), infection, and many other diseases.

The blood group is important in case blood transfusions are required and to plan future procedures if they become necessary.

- **Urine: Routine and Microscopic Examination**

  This is a detailed analysis of urine. It helps to detect any change in the composition of the urine, which helps in the diagnosis of many disorders.

- **Urine: Microalbumin**

  This checks the level of albumin in the urine. An above-normal level of albumin means your kidneys are stressed or have been damaged. Microalbuminuria is most often caused by kidney damage due to diabetes. However, many other conditions, such as high blood pressure, heart failure, cirrhosis, or lupus can lead to kidney damage.

Biochemistry Tests

The different body tissues release specific enzymes when they suffer damage. The biochemistry of the blood gives us an indication of what is happening within the body. Abnormal levels of specific enzymes help in localizing the problem. If certain organs are not eliminating certain waste products it indicates that they are not functioning properly.

- **Blood Glucose**

  Diet, liver function and how well the body is utilizing the glucose in the blood is indicated by the blood glucose levels. Excessively high glucose levels may be caused by diabetes mellitus; low values of blood sugar or hypoglycaemia can result from severe exertion or other conditions like pancreatic cancer or adrenal disease.

- **Lipid Profile**

  The lipid profile results are a good indicator of whether someone is likely to have a heart attack or stroke. The lipid profile includes total cholesterol, HDL-cholesterol (the good cholesterol), LDL-cholesterol (the bad cholesterol) and triglycerides. At times the report includes additional calculated results such as HDL/Cholesterol ratio or a risk score based on lipid profile, age, sex and other risk factors. If heart disease runs in the family, it is advisable to do a blood lipid profile in the late twenties and follow up with yearly or biennial checks depending on the result. The results help to plan treatment and follow-up for those at risk. The aim is to keep the total cholesterol and triglyceride levels on the lower side of the range, the HDL levels high and the LDL levels low.

- **Apolipoprotein A^1, B**

  Apolipoprotein A^1, a protein, carried in HDL (good) cholesterol helps remove bad types of cholesterol from the body. Along with the other lipid tests Apolipoprotein B levels are used to help determine an individual's risk of developing cardiovascular disease. This test can help to diagnose the cause of hyperlipidaemia, in someone who has elevated triglyceride levels. The latter can prevent accurate calculations of LDL cholesterol.

  Both an apo A-1 test which is associated with the HDL and an apo B test may be ordered to determine the apo B/apo A-1 ratio; which can be used to evaluate the risk of cardiovascular disease as an alternative to the total cholesterol/HDL ratio.

- **Blood Urea Nitrogen (BUN)**

  An end product of protein metabolism, urea is excreted by the kidneys. BUN levels increase in any condition that reduces kidney filtration rates or increases protein breakdown. Heart and circulatory conditions, which decrease blood flow to the kidneys, can increase BUN levels.

- **Lp(a)**

  The test for lipoprotein(a) while not a routine part of the lipid profiles is used to identify the presence of Lp(a) as a possible risk factor in the development of heart disease.

  Certain factors that can contribute to an elevated level of Lp(a) include a family history of high cholesterol levels, uncontrolled diabetes, severe hypothyroidism and certain renal conditions.

  The Lp(a) level is genetically determined. It remains relatively constant over an individual's lifetime. Lifestyle changes and most drugs do not affect it. As a result the Lp(a) is not the target of therapy. High Lp(a) is an added risk factor that suggests the need for aggressive treatment of the more treatable risk factors.

- **Serum Creatinine**

  The kidneys are responsible for eliminating creatinine, a waste product that originates from muscles. Creatinine levels can increase due to kidney disease or dehydration. Both creatinine and BUN increase in the bloodstream at the same time in patients with kidney disease.

- **Serum Uric Acid**

  Uric acid is created when the body breaks down purines from foods such as liver, beans and fish or from drinks such as wine and beer. The kidneys eliminate it from the blood and it is excreted in the urine. Diabetes may be one of the causes of elevated uric acid levels. Persons with elevated levels have an increased risk of developing kidney disease or gout.

- **Liver Function Tests**

  The liver as an organ has multiple functions. It is responsible for producing substances important for body functions like certain blood clotting factors and bile, the latter being very important in digestive and excretory functions. The different liver tests tell us how each component of the liver mechanism is functioning.

  - **Alanine Transaminase (ALT)** is a liver enzyme which speeds up chemical reactions. ALT levels usually rise when the liver is injured or inflamed (as in hepatitis).

  - **Aspartate Aminotransferase (AST)** is another enzyme which is usually found inside liver cells. When the levels are elevated it usually means the liver is injured in some way. Since the heart or skeletal muscle also releases ALT when damaged, AST is usually considered to be more specifically related to liver problems.

  - **Alkaline Phosphatase (ALP)** is an enzyme which is found mainly in liver cells next to bile ducts, and in bones. Its levels increase in some types of liver and bone diseases.

  - **Albumin**, the main protein produced in the liver, circulates in the bloodstream. The ability to produce albumin (and other proteins) is affected in some types of liver disorders, which result in a low level of albumin in the blood.

  - **Total protein** measures the levels of albumin and all other proteins in blood.

  - **Bilirubin** is a chemical which gives bile its yellow/green colour. A high level of bilirubin in the blood will make you jaundiced ('yellow'). It is the result of the breakdown of haemoglobin.

- **Homocysteine**

  It is a measure of the level of the amino acid homocysteine in the blood. It is one of the tests that help to identify the deficiency of Vitamin B12 or folic acid. It helps identify a rare inherited disorder 'homocystinuria' which results in a deficiency of one of several enzymes which help to convert food to energy. It may help determine the cause of unexplained blood clots.

  Elevated levels of homocysteine in the blood may be associated with atherosclerosis as also an increased risk for formation of blood clots, heart attacks, strokes and possibly Alzheimer's disease.

- **hs-CRP**

  The liver produces the C-Reactive Protein (CRP) when there is any inflammation in the body. It is suggested that there is a strong association between excessive inflammation and heart disease. Testing for hs-CRP is used as a way of predicting the risk of developing heart disease and its complications, namely heart attacks, disease of the peripheral vessels, stroke and sudden cardiac death. A higher hs-CRP level is linked to a higher risk of these problems.

- **Glycosylated Hb/Haemoglobin A1c Test/HbA1c**

  The haemoglobin A1c test is a blood test that is used to determine how well the blood sugar levels have been controlled over the last three-month period. It helps to maintain tight control by measuring long-term results.

  Haemoglobin is a blood molecule present in the red blood cells, which carries oxygen from the lungs to all other tissues of the body. When glucose attaches to haemoglobin a type of haemoglobin called haemoglobin A1c (HbA1c) forms. The higher the blood glucose level, the more the glycosylation of haemoglobin that will occur, resulting in a higher HbA1c level.

  The life of a red blood cell is approximately 120 days. There will always be a mixture of old and new red blood cells circulating in the bloodstream. The old cells would have been exposed to recent, and not so recent, blood glucose levels; while the new cells will only have been exposed to recent blood glucose levels. It is suggested that half of an HbA1c value is attributable to the previous month, a further quarter to the month prior to that, and the other quarter to the two months before that; this indirectly gives an idea of how well the blood sugar levels have been controlled over the last three months.

- **Thyroid Profile**

  The thyroid is a butterfly shaped gland located in the neck. It takes iodine from the blood and combines it with an amino acid to form thyroid hormones. Thyroxine, one of the hormones, is responsible for the metabolism. For individuals with almost any type of heart disease, thyroid gland disorders can worsen old cardiac symptoms or cause new ones, and can accelerate the underlying heart problem. Thyroid function tests, which commonly measure the T3, T4, TSH, free T3 and free T4 levels among others, help to determine whether the thyroid is functioning appropriately.

However, just blood tests are not enough to diagnose a cardiac problem. **Lung Function Tests** are non-invasive, diagnostic tests that provide feed-back about the functioning of the lung. Since these have a direct relation with the underlying cardiac status they may be adviced.

Now let us see why a chest X-Ray and further **Cardiac Evaluation** such as an ECG, Treadmill and other Stress Tests, and Echocardiography are needed to diagnose heart problems.

II. Cardiac Evaluation: A Case Scenario

Rakesh, aged 45 came to his cardiologist, for a follow up. Rakesh, a field executive, could not get over the fact that he had undergone a complete health check-up a month back, and had been told that he was hale and hearty, but a month later he had experienced severe chest pain and was rushed to hospital, where he was diagnosed as having suffered a heart attack!

At the time of his health check-up, his blood tests and ECG had been within normal limits. He therefore attributed the occasional discomfort he had been experiencing, to acidity.

His one burning question was, "Doctor, how did they miss my heart problem in the check-up?"

The doctor replied, "Well, the suspicion of heart blockages starts from the time we begin talking to our patient. We ask for symptoms, any medical history and obvious high risk factors, like a family history of heart disease, smoking, diabetes, high blood pressure and high cholesterol among others. Depending on the symptoms, tests are advised to rule out or confirm the problem."

"Doctor, I am a healthy 45-year-old, well I was (a wry grin), and my X-Ray and ECG were normal!"

The doctor said, "One needs to understand that for heart related issues a chest X-Ray can only show changes in the lungs stemming from heart problems or a change in the size and shape of the heart or any calcium present in the heart or blood vessels. A normal ECG does not mean no blockages. Unless a person is having an on going acute cardiac event or has had a previous major heart attack the resting ECG done during a regular check-up maybe normal in most cases. In fact in 15-20% of patients with a heart attack the ECG may be normal."

"What?" a little taken aback, Rakesh asked, "Doctor what is a stress test? Someone suggested that I would have probably known about my heart problem if I had undergone a stress test."

The doctor explained, "You need to understand that all the tests described can be performed under conditions of 'rest' or 'stress'. When you are lying down, relaxed it is a state of rest. When you run, get excited or climb stairs you drive the heart to work harder. The heart rate increases, more blood is required by the heart muscle to do its job and we say the heart is 'stressed'. Normally, when you exercise regularly the heart is 'conditioned' for that level of activity. Also when both the condition of the heart muscle and the blood vessels that supply it are good, the heart does not protest when we 'stress' it. No pain or discomfort is experienced.

However, in case the heart muscle cannot take the load or it does not receive enough blood it is likely to protest. There may be pain or discomfort, which could translate into a change in the ECG pattern.

A stress test pushes the heart to perform while detecting any signs of decreased blood supply to the heart. The person undergoing the test is made to exercise using a treadmill or cycle. For those unable to exercise for any reason, maybe orthopaedic problems, elderly people, debilitation, or chronic lung disease, non-exercise modalities are used. The latter is an artificial way of exercising the heart using different methods such as drugs like dobutamine, adenosine and dipyridamole, or atrial pacing, hyperventilation and afterload increase. The heart is an electrical pump. Different tests are needed to measure different aspects of its structure and working. The ECG or electrocardiogram only records the heart's electrical activity.

The echo or echocardiogram uses ultrasound waves to create images of the heart. It is a diagnostic test that helps to assess the health of both the heart chambers and the valves. The ability of the heart to pump the blood forward is also measured. But it cannot determine blockages in arteries from the heart. A normal echo does not mean that there are no blockages in the heart arteries.

Radiographic tests using X-Ray or other machines are carried out to create pictures of the internal structures of the chest.

New cardiac imaging techniques, such as cardiac Magnetic Resonance Imaging (MRI) and cardiac Computed Tomography (CT) allow the doctor to look more closely at the heart and great vessels with little risk to the patient."

The doctor continued, "There is a test, called the heart scan or the coronary calcium scan. It is a CT scan that measures the amount of calcium deposited in the heart arteries over the years, it only takes a couple of minutes. A coronary artery calcium score is then given. A positive scan tells us that the heart vessels are affected, but does not tell us how much of the vessel lumen is obstructed. The risks associated with the scan are low, although it does mean exposure to radiation, like any other radiological test."

Rakesh looked puzzled, "Doctor, if it does not tell me how much my arteries are blocked what is the use?"

The doctor said, "Here we are only trying to find out if there is a block in the heart arteries. The test is non-invasive, easily done and a calcium score of zero means you can relax. You are highly unlikely to have a block in the heart arteries. Depending on the calcium score your doctor would be able to advise medication or additional investigations if necessary, to exactly determine the blockages.

In fact, the coronary calcium scan is a useful diagnostic screening tool in certain situations. For example, if I have say a 20-year-old with a strong family history of diabetes, hypertension, heart disease who complains of chest pain on exertion. I would be inclined to suggest a coronary calcium scan. If the scan comes out clear, he can be advised that there is no underlying cardiac problem."

"That makes sense," Rakesh replied.

The doctor continued, "If one has to actually quantify the extent of blockages then we need to do a coronary angiography, still considered the gold standard to detect the health of the coronary arteries. In a coronary angiography a contrast dye is used to see an image of the blood vessels supplying the heart and assess how the heart is functioning. This is done by inserting a catheter into a blood vessel from the groin or the wrist directly into the coronary artery and injecting a dye. This is called cardiac catheterization. The dye is injected into the blood stream and a film of the heart is taken (Fig. 5).

The DynaCT is an angiography system that can rotate 360 degrees to provide CT-like images of the arteries. Because it requires less contrast agent, the DynaCT significantly reduces the patient's exposure to radiation while still providing an accurate diagnosis. Another test that may be carried out at the same time as the coronary angiography is the fractional flow reserve. A catheter is used to accurately measure flow past a blockage in a coronary artery.

Radioactive tracers like thallium or technetium are used to carry out a nuclear heart scan (also called radionuclide ventriculography or radionuclide imaging). The heart chambers and the major blood vessels that lead to and from the heart are delineated. Damage to the heart muscle can be seen. This test helps to diagnose heart disease, disorders of the blood vessels, or heart failure.

Three-dimensional pictures of the tissues inside the body can be recreated, using radioactive tracers by Positron Emission Tomography (PET) or a cardiac viability study. This is especially useful in patients who are unable to exercise, either on a treadmill or a stationary cycle. It helps to assess whether the heart muscle is receiving sufficient blood flow, and tells us how much the heart has been damaged after a heart attack, while also helping us to decide whether our treatment plan is effective or not. It is the gold standard way to assess how much of the heart muscle is viable in patients who have poor pumping. It helps us understand if the patient is likely to benefit from either an angioplasty or a bypass surgery.

As I explained earlier, both an ECG as well as nuclear scanning can be carried out after the heart is 'stressed'. This increases both the sensitivity and specificity of the test results.

An ECG stress test or a treadmill stress test is less expensive as compared to imaging techniques. It can assist in confirming the diagnosis, assessing the functioning of the heart and telling us how things are likely to be.

Stress echocardiography, is a well-tolerated and valuable procedure which helps to detect decreased blood flow to the heart muscle when it is stressed.

The stress thallium myocardial perfusion scintigraphy is a novel diagnostic tool. It helps to detect and determine the amount and status of heart muscle that is alive or dead. After stress, different areas of the heart show a difference in blood flow. The areas, which do not show an increase in flow, suggest that these areas are supplied by blood vessels, which have significant blockages.

This helps us to plan the appropriate management - angioplasty, surgery, medical management, stem cell therapy or rarely even a cardiac transplant.

In certain situations where an angiography misses a block, the stress thallium perfusion scan will pick up a perfusion defect With the addition of more refined and newer compounds like Technetium, the nuclear perfusion test offers more details and additional information like the pumping rate of the heart, heart muscle contractility and movement of the various walls of the heart.

It must be remembered that all tests have limitations. At times in order to reach a definite conclusion, additional tests maybe suggested," the doctor stressed.

Rakesh was thoughtful, "Doctor, you are saying that I may have had regular blood tests, the ECG maybe normal and I could still end up with a heart attack. That is scary. Is it not possible to diagnose a block in the heart arteries before an attack actually takes place? I mean I am only 45-years-old, I have regular medical check-ups, no symptoms and no 'bad' habits." After a pause he added, "Well I do have a family history."

The doctor nodded, "Unless we have someone actually complaining of symptoms, showing up an abnormality in the ECG or other cardiac evaluation tests we would not be inclined to advise an angiography. But as I explained, in view of your family history we could probably have done a coronary calcium scan."

Rakesh shook the doctor's hand, thanked him and left the consulting room, thinking that indeed, more than a couple of tests are needed to diagnose heart disease. And just knowing the names of tests to be done was not enough. One needed to understand what the results mean.

III. Know Your Basic Numbers

Just knowing what tests to undergo is not enough. You have to understand what the results mean. The doctor will look at the results when you visit him/her and advise you accordingly. It is important to look after yourself and monitor your health on a regular basis. Today, with home care products like automatic blood pressure apparatus and glucometers, more and more individuals are checking themselves to ensure tight control over their risk factors.

BMI or Body Mass Index

The Body Mass Index (BMI) is a calculation that uses your height and weight to estimate how much body fat you have.

- English BMI Formula:

  BMI = (Weight in pounds/(Height in inches)^2 x 703
- Metric BMI Formula:

  BMI = (Weight in kilograms/(Height in metres)^2

A person with a higher BMI is thought to be at a greater risk of heart disease, diabetes and other weight-related problems.

A calculation of your BMI will help you to understand in which category you fall: underweight, healthy weight, overweight or obese.

BMI Categories

Classification	BMI
Underweight	≤ 18.5
Healthy weight	18.5-24.9
Overweight	25-29.9
Obesity	≥ 30

Your overall health and well-being depend on reaching and maintaining a healthier weight. Even losing a few kilograms or preventing further weight gain has health benefits in the obese individual.

Blood Pressure

Normal blood pressure in a healthy adult is below 120/80 mm Hg. The top number is the force generated when the heart pumps the blood and the bottom number is when the heart is relaxed.

When the heart beats, the blood is pumped into the vessels called arteries, which form a network that distributes the blood to all parts of your body. Blood pressure is the force of the blood pushing against the walls of the arteries. Every time the heart beats (normally about 60-70 times a minute at rest) it pumps out blood into the arteries. Your blood pressure is at its highest when the heart beats, pumping the blood forward. This is called the systolic pressure. When the heart is at rest, between beats, blood pressure falls. This is the diastolic pressure.

Blood pressure is measured by recording these two values, the systolic and diastolic pressures. Both are important. The value of the blood pressure is written as 120/80 mm Hg.

Blood pressure varies with activity; it may be high when a person is under any kind of stress (physical or mental) and in the normal range when a person is at rest or mentally at ease.

Continuous high blood pressure over a period of time can lead to heart disease. Often, persons with high blood pressure have no symptoms. This makes it all the more necessary for you to have your blood pressure checked routinely and take any medicine that is advised regularly.

The blood pressure categories as defined by the American Heart Association are:

Blood Pressure Category	Systolic (mmHg)/Diastolic (mmHg)		
Normal	< 120	and	< 80
Prehypertension	120-139	or	80-89
High Blood Pressure (Hypertension) Stage 1	140-159	or	90-99
High Blood Pressure (Hypertension) Stage 2	> 160	or	> 100
Hypertensive Crisis (Emergency care needed)	> 180	or	> 110

Cholesterol and Triglyceride Levels

Individuals with high levels of cholesterol and/or triglycerides in the blood may not suffer from any symptoms. It is important to get both levels checked regularly. If the levels are found to be high, your doctor may advise medication along with a diet and exercise regime targeted to reducing the cholesterol and triglyceride levels.

Total Cholesterol	
< 200 mg/dL	Desirable
200-239 mg/dL	Borderline High
> 240 mg/dL	High

LDL (Bad) Cholesterol	
< 100 mg/dL	Desirable
100-129 mg/dL	Near Desirable
130-159 mg/dL	Borderline High
160-189 mg/dL	High
> 190	Very High

HDL (Good) Cholesterol	
< 40 mg/dL	Carries major risk for heart disease
40-59 mg/dL	Higher the better
> 60 mg/dL	Protective against heart disease

Triglycerides	
< 150 mg/dL	Normal
150-199 mg/dL	Borderline high
200-499 mg/dL	High
> 500 mg/dL	Very High

Source: National Heart, Lung and Blood Institute

Blood Sugar Levels

Often persons with high blood glucose have no symptoms. Blood glucose should be checked regularly. Your doctor will decide what form and dosage of medication you need. It could be pills or insulin injections. A healthy diet and exercise plan would also be suggested.

Blood sugar values are reported in units of mg/dl or mmol/L depending on the laboratory or device used.

Result	Fasting Plasma Glucose	Value 2 hours after consuming glucose
Normal	< 100 mg/dL	< 140 mg/dL
Prediabetes 125 mg/dL	100 mg/dL to to 199 mg/dL	140 mg/dL
Diabetes or higher	126 mg/dL	200 mg/dL or higher

Source: American Diabetes Association

Diabetes Control Chart
HbA1c

Test score	Interpretation
< 9.0-14.0	Poor control
< 7.0-9.0	Good control
4.0-7.0	Excellent control

Mean Blood Glucose (mg/dL)	Interpretation
< 215	Poor control
150-180	Good control
50-115	Excellent Control

According to the Diabetes Control and Complications Trial (DCCT) conducted from 1983 to 1993 and the follow-up study, Epidemiology of Diabetes Interventions and Complications (EDIC), for every point that the A1C levels are lowered the risk of developing a variety of complications is also lowered:

- Risk of eye disease is reduced by 76 per cent.
- Risk of kidney disease is reduced by 50 per cent.
- Risk of nerve disease is reduced by 60 per cent.
- The risk of any cardiovascular disease is reduced by 42 per cent.
- Risk of a nonfatal heart attack, stroke, or risk of death from cardiovascular causes is reduced by 57 per cent.

If you have been diagnosed with diabetes you should check your blood glucose levels frequently. The glucose levels should be tested before and after meals to see how eating affects them.

In order to lower your HbA1c, you need a better picture of how your blood sugar changes throughout the day, as there may be periods of time when your blood sugar maybe high without your knowing it.

Chapter 4

Managing Coronary Artery Disease

I. Procedures and Therapies

Preview - What Are We Looking At?

Who should get tested? What tests should be performed? Who should be treated for coronary artery disease and how to treat them? These have always been questions of debate. The questions are probably the result of lack of consensus between the 'old school of thought' and 'the new school of thought' about what coronary artery disease really is.

The Old School of Thought

The old school of thought subscribes to the fact that blockages in the coronary artery cause angina and then a heart attack. The final aim is to relieve the block. The primary focus is to determine the exact position of the blockage and quantify the degree and number of blockages. The traditional thinkers believe that cardiac catheterization is the only appropriate way to diagnose any blockages and that angioplasty or stenting, and somewhat reluctantly cardiac bypass surgery, are considered the only possible treatment options.

The New School of Thought

It is now known that coronary artery disease is in fact a chronic condition, which progresses over time. Coronary arteries may be characterized by the presence of plaques or there could be generalized narrowing of the coronary arteries present with or without blockages. Rupture of plaque may precipitate the formation of a blood clot in the artery causing an acute blockage resulting in chest pain or a heart attack. The new way of thinking considers the presence of plaques as a way of diagnosing coronary artery disease.

Do We Need to Think Further?

Blockages hamper blood flow, and blood clots obstruct blood flow as does constriction of the arteries. Collaterals are natural bypasses that develop around areas of blood flow obstruction as seen in people who exercise; they seem to improve blood flow and reduce symptoms. The collateral vessels, although much smaller than the main coronary arteries, still manage to deliver enough oxygen and nutrients to the heart muscle.

This seems to suggest that obstructions or blockages are just causes that reduce the blood flow; it is finally the amount of blood flow to the heart muscle that decides whether a person will suffer from a heart attack or not.

The treatment of coronary artery disease therefore requires aggressive correction of any risk factors and an intensive medical therapy. The final aim being to improve blood flow in the coronary arteries by:

- Preventing new blockages.
- Reversing old blockages when possible.
- Keeping the inner lining of the coronary arteries smooth.
- Stabilizing the plaques.
- Preventing the formation of blood clots.

All aspects of prevention, treatment and management do one or more of the above. They essentially work to maintain the blood flow to the heart muscle. Finally, whatever measure is used, the determining factor is how much the blood supply to the heart has increased.

Treatment Options

If the blocks in the coronary arteries are left untreated, they progress over time and cause ongoing damage to the heart muscle and a threat to life. The treatment modalities available include medication, medical therapies, surgical intervention or Percutaneous Coronary Intervention (PCI). The treatment interventions are aimed at relieving the blocks, improving the blood flow to the heart muscle and relieving any conditions that occur as a result of the blockages. Some of these are temporary procedures that may be adopted in a hospital setting to improve coronary artery flow, while the others are used as treatment options.

1. Coronary Angioplasty

• Coronary Balloon Angioplasty

Introduced in the late 1970s, balloon angioplasty or Percutaneous Transluminal Coronary Angioplasty (PTCA), also called Percutaneous Coronary Intervention (PCI), is a non-surgical procedure. It relieves narrowing and obstruction of the arteries to the muscle of the heart.

The procedure is conducted in a cardiac catheterization laboratory. Routinely done under local anesthesia, a thin, flexible catheter (tube) with a balloon at its tip is threaded through a peripheral blood vessel, the femoral artery in the groin or the radial artery at the wrist, to the affected artery. The position of the catheter is determined by imaging techniques. Once in place, the balloon is inflated to compress the plaque against the artery wall. This restores the blood flow through the artery.

• Coronary Angioplasty with Stents

During the coronary angioplasty, the blockages can be dilated and mechanical devices called stents are left at the site of the blockage. The stents act as scaffolds to hold the artery open (Fig. 6). This treats the focal area of narrowing, thus relieving the obstruction. The stent used for scaffolding the coronary artery maybe a bare metal stent or a drug eluting stent.

The bare metal stents have a wire mesh design, which allows the stent to be collapsed when it is being deployed. Once in place it opens up to match the artery wall configuration. Over time the inner artery wall tends to eventually grow over the stent.

The bare metal stents can be *drug eluting*; which means that the stent is medicated. The medication is released over a period of time. This allows the medication to be repeatedly released to the area where the stent is placed, thus preventing the vessel from clogging up again and at the same time helping to prevent clotting.

- **The Risks**

  The possible risks are associated with the stents *per se* and the procedure. During the procedure the coronary artery can be damaged or ruptured. There could be an allergic reaction either to the stent or the medication on the stent, or a blood clot at the stent site.

  After the stent is placed it will be recommended that the individual take blood thinning and anti-clotting medication to reduce these risks. It is important to take these medications as advised and directed for the prescribed period.

2. Atherectomy

Considering that plaque is at the root of the problem, as it blocks the coronary arteries, different plaque removal or atherectomy devices were developed as adjuncts to PCI. A laser catheter or a rotating shaver can be used.

Photoablation is the use of light or a laser to destroy tissue. The excimer laser is used for photoablation of plaque.

- **Directional atherectomy** is where the plaque is cut and removed (Fig. 7.1).
- **Rotational atherectomy** uses a high-speed diamond-encrusted drill to mechanically ablate the plaque (Fig. 7.2).

Initially believed to decrease restenosis incidence, it has now been shown that atherectomy is of little additional benefit. Atherectomy is now employed as an adjunct to PCI in select cases.

3. Brachytherapy

Brachytherapy or internal radiotherapy uses beta radiation to open the blocked heart arteries. The radiation in coronary artery brachytherapy prevents cells from reproducing and causing blockage of the coronary artery. It is usually used as an adjunct to angioplasty and stent placement.

4. Transmyocardial Laser Revascularisation (TMLR)

In a certain group of people suffering from coronary artery disease it may not be possible to offer an angioplasty or a surgical option. Instead Transmyocardial Laser Revascularization (TMLR), a type of surgery, can be offered. It cannot cure CAD, but it may reduce the pain of angina. In this procedure a high powered carbon dioxide or other laser is used to make tiny channels both through the heart muscle and the left ventricle – the heart's main pumping chamber. When the oxygen-rich blood enters the left ventricle, blood flowing through the channels will carry much-needed oxygen to the deprived heart muscle.

The process is probably likely to have two beneficial effects, the procedure may help angiogenesis, i.e., the heart muscle grows new blood vessels and another school of thought supports the view that the TMLR laser destroys some of the pain-causing nerves in the heart muscle.

The positive effects of denervation added to the increased blood flow occurring over time may make TMLR a successful therapy.

The idea originated from a study of alligator and snake hearts where the heart muscle receives oxygen and nutrition directly from the ventricle and not through the coronary arteries.

5. Enhanced External Counter Pulsation (EECP)

Enhanced External Counter Pulsation is a non-invasive technique that does not require surgery, needles or medication.

EECP improves the balance between the oxygen requirement and oxygen supply of the heart. The aim is to increase oxygen-rich blood flow to the heart and reduce the heart's workload. EECP uses timed, sequential inflation of pressure cuffs on the legs.

The individual undergoing EECP, is fitted with pneumatic stockings/pressure cuffs on their legs; three cuffs are placed on each leg (on the calf, the lower thigh, and the upper thighs (or buttock)). The heart rate and rhythm are monitored using telemetry monitors. The cuffs are timed to inflate and deflate based on the individual's electrocardiogram. The cuffs should ideally inflate at the beginning of the relaxation phase of the heart and deflate at the beginning of the contraction phase of the heart. During the inflation portion of the cycle, the calf cuffs inflate first, then the lower thigh cuffs and finally the upper thigh cuffs. The inflation are controlled by a pressure monitor.

When inflated, the pressure cuffs on the leg gently compress the blood vessels in the legs forcing blood back to the heart (Fig. 8).

As a result:

- The pressure the heart must pump against is lowered.
- The rate of return of blood to the heart increases.
- The blood pressure increases when the heart is resting.

EECP treatment is not a substitute for other treatments but can be used in conjunction with other medical therapies and recommendations.

6. Coronary Artery Bypass Surgery

This is a surgical way of fixing blocks. In the surgical technique, the blocks are generally not touched. A detour, using another blood vessel, is created around the block just as a detour is set up when there is a road block (Fig. 9.1) and (Fig. 9.2) respectively.

Coronary bypass surgery is described as being on-pump and off-pump surgery.

- **On Pump Coronary Artery Surgery**

  The coronary arteries run on the surface of the heart. To allow the surgeon to operate on them the heart is rested. The blood flow through the heart is diverted to a heart-lung machine, which as the name suggests serves the function of both the heart and the lungs i.e., it maintains the circulation and oxygenates the blood as it passes through the machine (Fig. 10). This allows the heart to be emptied and also rests the lungs. The surgeon can complete the procedure on a quiet heart. Once the surgery is completed, the heart and lungs are gradually allowed to take over their normal function.

- **Off Pump Coronary Artery Surgery**

  In off pump surgery the surgeon works on the surface of the heart while the heart continues to beat and the lungs continue to carry out their normal respiratory functions. The surgeon 'stabilizes' the heart using stabilizing devices like the Octopus (OctoEvo) and the Starfish (Fig. 11)   and

(Fig. 12) respectively. The octopus has vacuum cups, which allow it to rest on the heart, relatively immobilizing the portion of the heart that is being operated upon.

- **The Detour**

  The detour is created using another blood vessel, either a vein or an artery.

  Traditionally the saphenous vein from the leg is used as a vessel for the bypass. The graft vessels are sewn to the coronary arteries beyond the narrowing or blockage. The other end of this vein is attached to the aorta (the main artery that leaves the heart).

  Other arteries used for the bypass are the artery in the forearm called the radial artery, the arteries that run on the inside of the chest wall called the internal thoracic arteries or the internal mammary arteries and rarely the gastroepiploic artery.

  The radial artery graft is easy to prepare and was used in the early years of coronary surgery. The long-term results of radial artery grafts suggest that the results are not as good as those when the Internal Thoracic Arteries (ITAs) are used as grafts.

  There are two internal thoracic arteries, one on either side of the sternum (breast bone). One advantage of using these arteries is that no additional incision has to be made anywhere else on the body. The entire surgery can be done through one incision.

  The left ITA is left attached at its origin and the free right internal thoracic artery is connected like a 'Y'. The two are then connected along the course of the coronary arteries beyond the blocks. These arteries tend to remain patent longer than venous grafts.

  Another artery the Gastroepiploic Artery (GEA), a branch of the artery that supplies blood to the stomach can also be used as a bypass graft usually to the right coronary artery, however, it is a technically difficult operation to perform and so has not become a popular bypass graft.

  In certain patients, instead of a total venous (all vein grafts) or a total arterial (all arterial grafts) technique, a hybrid approach may be adopted. One arterial and one or two vein grafts or two arterial and one vein graft or other permutations are employed.

The decision as to what kind of graft to use for the detour is determined by the surgeon performing the operation. Sometimes, the initial surgical plan may change depending on what is found during the surgery.

- **Approaches**

  The heart can be approached in different ways during the surgery. In a mid-sternotomy approach the breast bone (sternum) is slit down the middle and the heart, which lies just below it, is easily accessed.

  In Minimally Invasive Cardiac Surgery (MICS), Coronary Artery Bypass Grafting (CABG), keyhole surgery or the McGinn technique, the coronary bypass is carried out through several small incisions rather than the traditional median sternotomy. It is a beating heart procedure that is performed through an opening on the side of the thoracic wall.

  Totally Endoscopic, Minimally Invasive Coronary Artery Bypass (TECAB) is an advanced form of MICAS surgery. It uses a surgical robot to perform the bypass through three or four small holes in the chest cavity through which the two robotic arms and one camera are inserted.

  Certain centres may adopt the hybrid technique and combine a minimally invasive bypass surgery and stented angioplasty in one operation.

- **Life of the graft**

  All surgeons would like to promise the patient that the grafts will never have to be redone. Unfortunately, in reality, the situation is more complex. Anyone who undergoes a bypass surgery has certain risk factors, some of which will continue even after the surgery is performed. If the natural course of the disease progresses, then over time the original coronary artery can suffer new blocks, and any existing smaller plaques may increase in size. At times, the conduits, which have been used, may themselves be affected and not be of good quality. This will cause blockages to occur within the grafts themselves.

Pacemakers

There may be occasions, when due to the blocks in the coronary arteries, the electrical system of the heart may be affected causing problems in the rhythm. When the heart slows down, sufficient blood is not ejected and so the organs are affected. An 'artificial pacemaker' is then used to send electrical impulses to restore the heart's regular rhythm. The electrical impulses are sent to the heart using an electrode, which is placed next to the heart wall.

An artificial pacemaker can replace a defective natural pacemaker or blocked pathway. Some pacemakers are permanently (internal) implanted in the body and some are temporary (external) (Fig. 13.1) and (Fig. 13.2) respectively. A temporary pacemaker helps to tide over an acute crisis.

The pacemaker can be a standard pacemaker that triggers the heart chambers. The pacing system typically comprises a pacemaker, one or two leads, and a programmer. When the rhythm of the heart is irregular or too slow the pacemaker sends tiny electrical impulses that pace the heart. The pacing lead, an insulated wire, carries the impulse from the pacemaker to the heart assisting it to beat. A programme is used to set the way the impulses are to be generated and conducted.

The second type, the internal defibrillator/pacemaker combination is known as a cardioverter defibrillator. Like a standard pacemaker it sends an electrical impulse to the heart to control the heart's rate and rhythm and is also additionally programmed to deliver a 'shock' to stop a rhythm that can be fatal. It senses when the rhythm turns critical and delivers a pre-programmed shock to restore a normal stable rhythm.

All coronary artery blockages do not require an intervention. They can be managed with medicines.

II. Medical Management

It must be remembered that any drug that has 'effects' will also have some side effects. It is vital that all drugs are taken as prescribed by your doctor. The medications and dosages will be adjusted according to your needs and the other drugs prescribed.

Modern day management of CAD has a number of goals, namely increased survival; reduction in the atherosclerotic process in the coronary arteries; a reduction in myocardial necrosis, thereby preventing dysfunction of the left ventricle and left ventricle remodelling, preventing the onset of new and acute coronary syndrome; and most importantly improving the Quality of Life (QoL) of the patient.

The drugs used in management of CAD are discussed below.

1. Anticoagulants

Anticoagulants although described as blood thinning medicines do not actually thin the blood. They essentially increase the time that the blood needs to clot. This prevents an increase in the size of any existing clot thereby preventing a heart attack or even a stroke. They are used to prevent blood clots from forming in the heart during or after a heart attack. Anticoagulants may also be given following an angioplasty to prevent the formation of a new clot after the procedure.

Anticoagulants are very effective. In patients who have had a heart attack they reduce the rate of suffering a stroke or a recurrent heart attack. In patients with unstable angina or who have recently undergone an angioplasty with or without stenting, anticoagulants may lessen the risk of a heart attack. In patients who have suffered a major heart attack on the front wall of the heart, anticoagulants reduce the risk of a stroke.

Examples of anticoagulants that may be advised are:

- Unfractionated heparins: Heparin.
- Low Molecular Weight Heparins (LMWH): Fragmin or Lovenox.
- Coumarins: Warfarin (Coumadin).
- Direct thrombin inhibitors (generally only used in hospital settings): Bivalirudin, Fondaparinux, Lepirudin.

As expected, bleeding is the most common side effect of anticoagulants. If you are taking the medication then it is vital that you consult your doctor in case of any new bruises, a nosebleed that does not stop quickly, bleeding gums, blood in the urine, streaks of blood in your stools or black coloured stools, heavy menstrual bleeding or bleeding in between your periods.

Persons taking Warfarin need to undergo regular blood tests, eat a proper diet and know which foods can interact with the medication causing the level of Warfarin in the blood to increase or decrease.

It is also important to tell your dentist or doctor that you are taking anticoagulant medication, if you have to undergo a surgical procedure. They may need to stop the medication a few days prior to the procedure or change to another form of anticoagulant depending on the risks and requirements.

2. Aspirin

Aspirin has two main actions on the body:

- Anti-prostaglandin and anti-inflammatory: reducing fever and relieving pain.
- Anti-platelet, 'blood thinning' action.

The anti-platelet action prevents the formation of blood clots in the arteries. It reduces the chances of a heart attack or stroke, especially if you have risk factors like high blood pressure, smoking, high cholesterol or diabetes.

It is suggested that one should take aspirin during a heart attack. It slows the blood clotting and reduces the severity of the heart attack.

Low-dose aspirin may be suggested:

- For those with coronary artery disease.
- Following a heart attack, to prevent another one.
- For those suffering from stable or unstable angina.
- Following a bypass surgery or angioplasty.
- For those who have suffered a stroke or transient ischemic attack.
- For healthy men over 45 years of age and women over 55 years of age.

While daily aspirin can benefit both men and women who have never suffered from a heart attack or a stroke, the benefits differ according to gender. For men, aspirin seems to work better in preventing a heart attack, while in women it seems to work better in preventing a stroke.

For those with a history of a previous heart attack or stroke, aspirin can help prevent a second attack.

3. Clopidogrel Bisulphate

Clopidogrel also has anti-platelet action. It keeps the blood from clotting to prevent unwanted blood clots. It is used to prevent blood clots after a recent heart attack or stroke, and is prescribed to people with certain disorders of the heart or blood vessels.

Enzymes in the liver activate clopidogrel to its active form. Those with reduced activity of the liver enzymes may not adequately respond to clopidogrel.

A dual anti-platelet therapy of aspirin and thienopyridines (clopidogrel or prasugrel) may be advised after placement of coronary stents to prevent thrombotic complications. The effectiveness of the combination is being further studied.

A word of caution: Antithrombotics should never be stopped without consulting the prescribing physician. Also any untoward bleeding incidents must be immediately reported to the consulting physician.

4. Thrombolytics

Thrombolysis is the therapeutic breakdown of a thrombus or blood clot. The emergence of thrombolytic or fibrinolytic drugs in the treatment of acute heart attacks and ischemic strokes subsequently parallels the history of the 'reperfusion' theory. It was found that clots caused blockages in the blood vessels resulting in tissue damage due to decreased forward blood flow to the organ or tissue. Dissolving these clots early *in vivo*, re-established and restored the blood flow to the organ and tissues thereby reducing the degree of subsequent damage.

Thrombolytic drugs include:

- Tissue plasminogen activator t-PA: Altepase, Reteplase, Tenecteplase.

- Anistreplase.
- Streptokinase.
- Urokinase.

The drugs are most effective if they are administered immediately after a clinical need for them is felt. Administered within 60 minutes of a thrombotic event the effect is maximum, but they can still be effective even if they are administered up to six hours after the onset of symptoms.

These drugs may be used in combination with other anticoagulant drugs like low molecular weight heparin, to enhance their synergistic antithrombotic effects and secondary prevention.

5. Glycoprotein IIb/IIIa receptor inhibitors

Platelets are central to the pathogenesis of atherosclerosis and the development of acute thrombotic events. Damage to the vessels' endothelium results in platelets adhering at the site. They are activated and secrete factors causing platelets to clump together and interact with the factors responsible for forming plaques and clots.

The glycoprotein IIb/IIIa or integrin complex found on platelets is instrumental in triggering platelet aggregation. The glycoprotein IIb/IIIa receptor inhibitor binds the circulatory clotting factors that crosslink platelets as the final pathway to platelet aggregation.

This group of drugs has been used to treat various coronary artery diseases.

6. Nitrates

Nitrates are vasodilators, i.e., medications that result in enlarging the blood vessels. They dilate the arteries of the heart, increasing blood flow to the heart and relieving any chest pain or discomfort. They dilate the veins throughout the body resulting in more blood being accommodated in the periphery. The amount of blood being brought back to the heart decreases. This in turn reduces the load on the heart.

It is not unusual for a person with a coronary artery disease to carry a nitrate in their wallet/purse. The most common types of

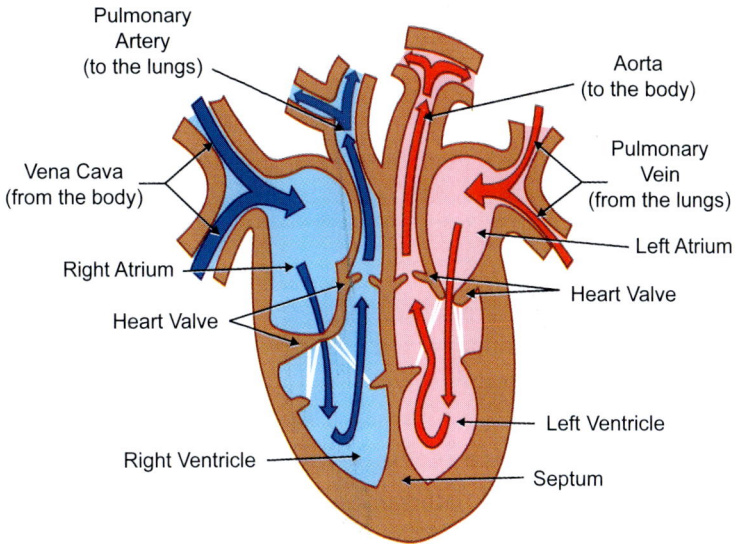

Fig. 1: Heart as a pump

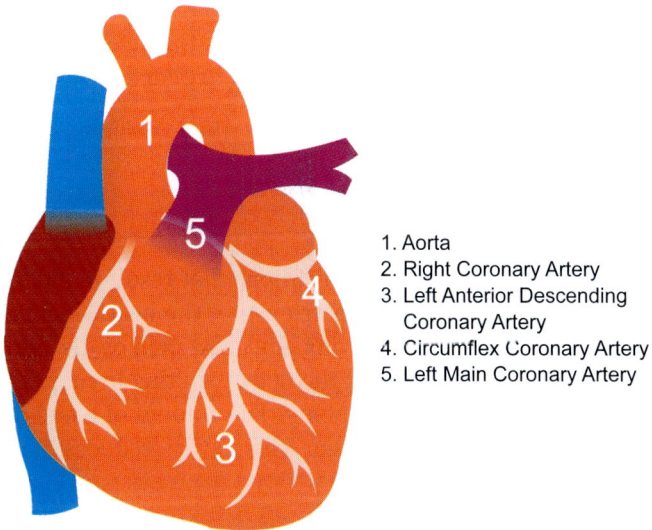

1. Aorta
2. Right Coronary Artery
3. Left Anterior Descending Coronary Artery
4. Circumflex Coronary Artery
5. Left Main Coronary Artery

Fig. 2: Coronary arteries

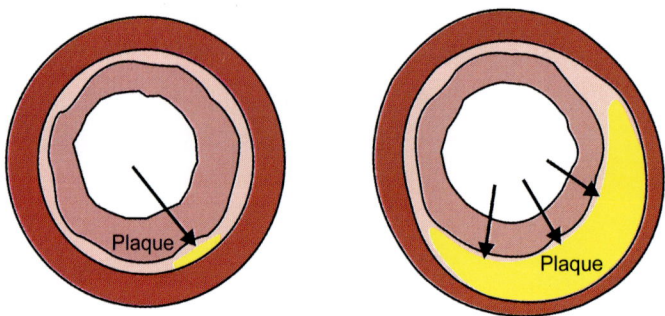

Fig. 3: Plaque build-up

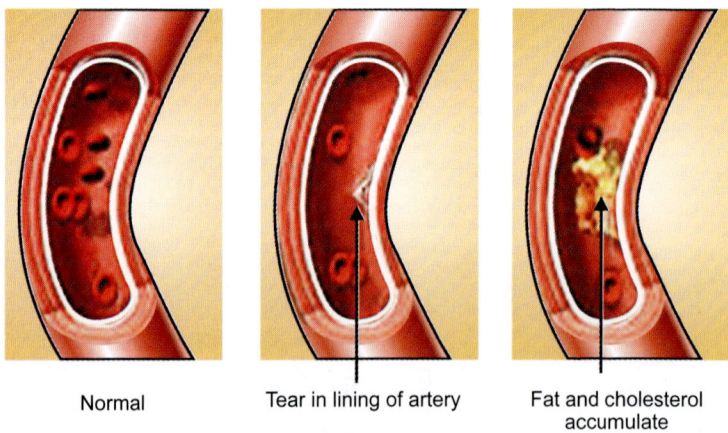

Normal

Tear in lining of artery

Fat and cholesterol accumulate

Fig. 4: Plaque build-up in coronary artery

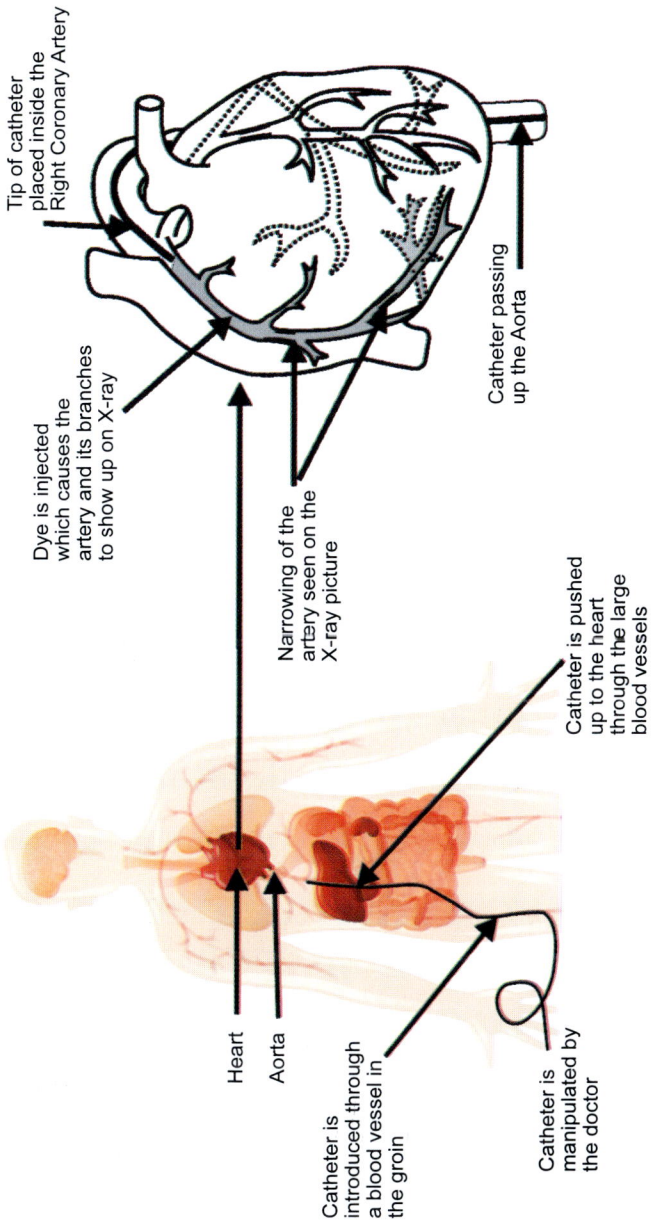

Tip of catheter placed inside the Right Coronary Artery

Dye is injected which causes the artery and its branches to show up on X-ray

Narrowing of the artery seen on the X-ray picture

Catheter passing up the Aorta

Heart

Aorta

Catheter is introduced through a blood vessel in the groin

Catheter is pushed up to the heart through the large blood vessels

Catheter is manipulated by the doctor

Fig. 5: Coronary angiography

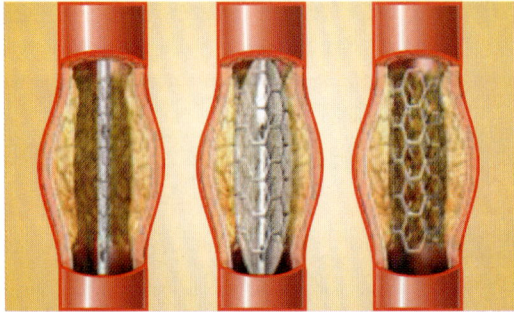

Stent inserted · Stent expanded · Stent stays in coronary artery

Fig. 6: Stent insertion

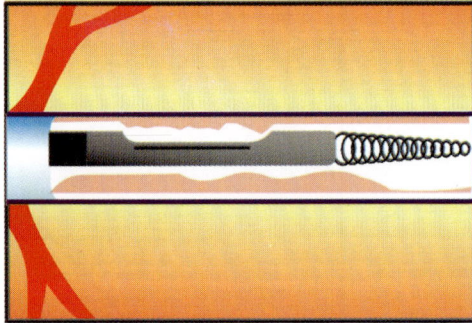

Fig. 7.1: Directional atherectomy device cuts and shaves away the plaque before removing it

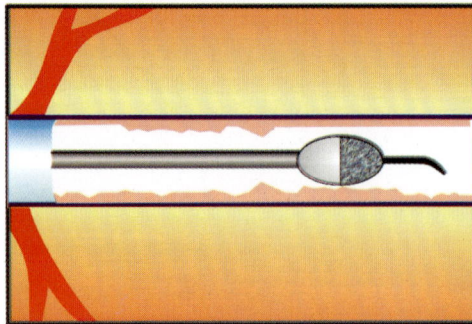

Fig. 7.2: Rotational atherectomy device goes through the plaque with a rotating blade

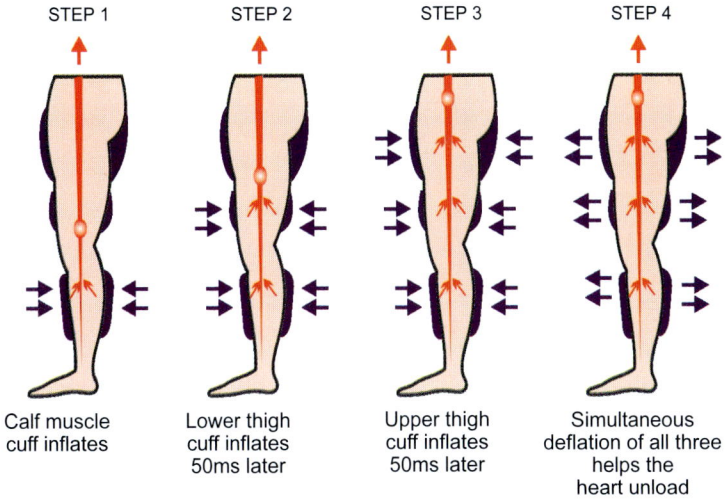

STEP 1 — Calf muscle cuff inflates

STEP 2 — Lower thigh cuff inflates 50ms later

STEP 3 — Upper thigh cuff inflates 50ms later

STEP 4 — Simultaneous deflation of all three helps the heart unload

Fig. 8: Effects of EECP on circulation

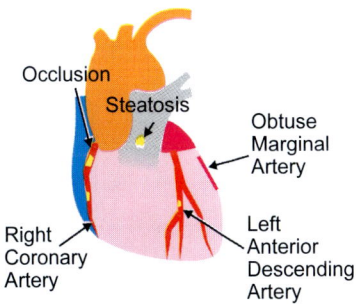

Occlusion

Steatosis

Obtuse Marginal Artery

Right Coronary Artery

Left Anterior Descending Artery

Fig. 9.1: Simplified view of the diseased heart before bypass surgery

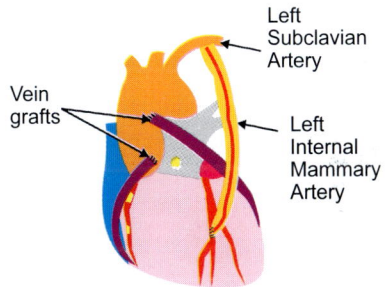

Left Subclavian Artery

Vein grafts

Left Internal Mammary Artery

Fig. 9.2: Simplified view of the heart after bypass surgery

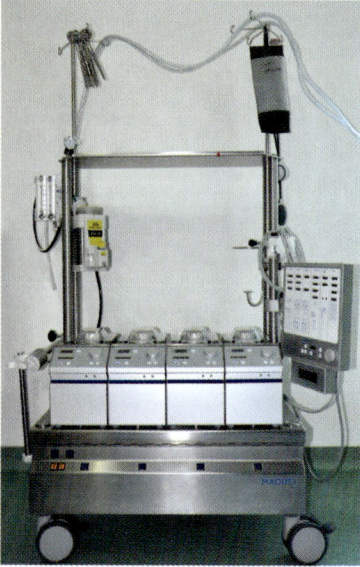

Fig. 10: Heart-Lung machine

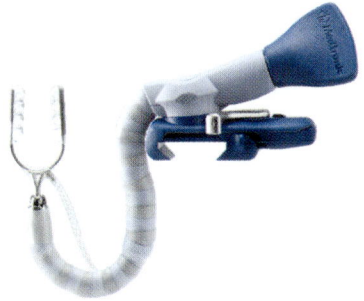

Fig. 11: OctoEvo

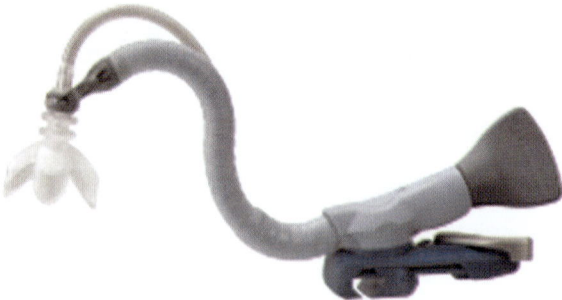

Fig. 12: Starfish

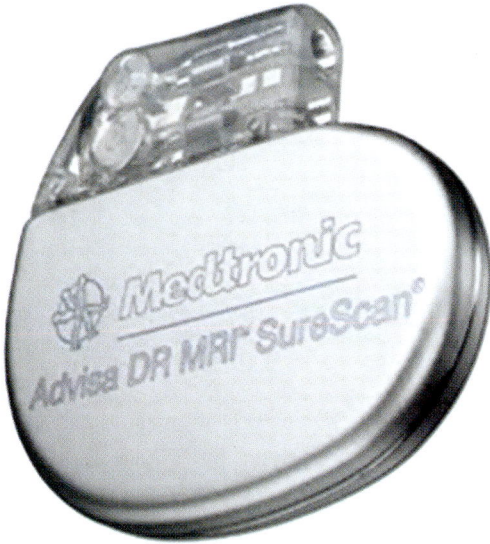

Fig. 13.1: Permanent pacemaker

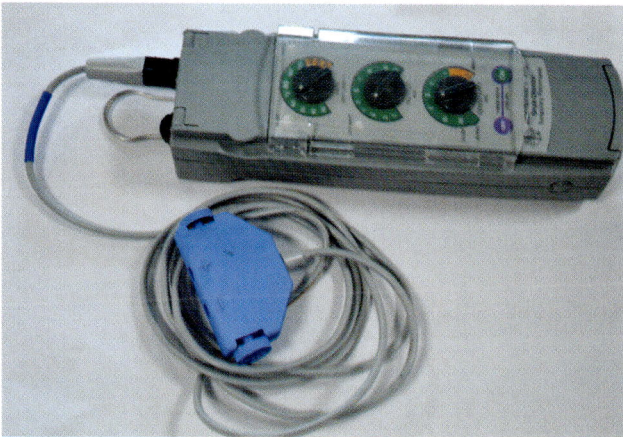

Fig. 13.2: Temporary pacemaker

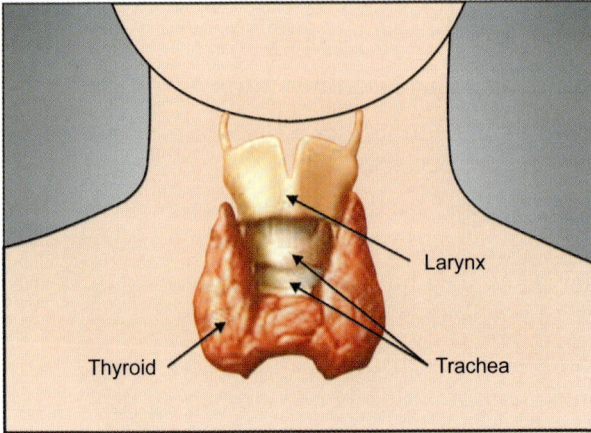

Fig. 14: Thyroid

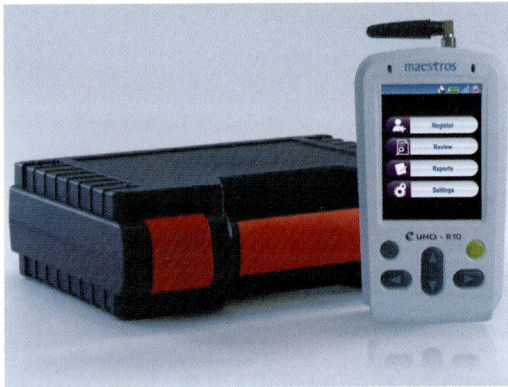

Fig. 15: Telecardiology solution

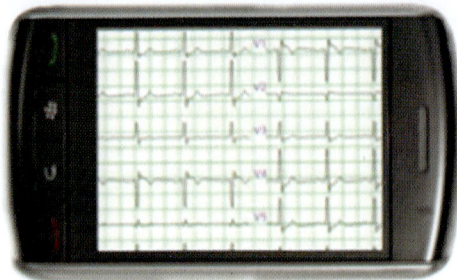

Fig. 16: ECG on mobile device

nitrates are nitroglycerin (Glyceryl Trinitrate (GTN)), isosorbide dinitrate, and isosorbide mononitrate.

They are used to treat angina in three ways:

- It is advised to take nitrates for a short-term on an 'as needed basis' to relieve angina.

- Short-term nitrates are to be taken prior to undertaking activities known to cause an angina attack.

- In certain cases long-term nitrate usage on a daily basis is suggested to reduce the number of angina attacks.

Since the nitrates cause dilation of the blood vessels, they can lead to complaints of headache, or dizziness due to a fall in blood pressure.

7. Angiotensin Converting Enzyme (ACE) Inhibitors and Angiotensin Receptor Blockers (ARBs)

Angiotensin Converting Enzyme inhibitors (ACEi) and Angiotensin Receptor Blockers (ARBs) are two classes of antihypertensive drugs. They act on the renin-angiotensin-aldosterone system, a hormonal system that regulates the blood pressure and the water balance of the body.

The liver releases angiotensinogen. When the volume of blood is low, rennin is secreted directly into the circulatory system by certain cells in the kidneys. This converts the angiotensinogen into angiotensin I, which is further, converted to angiotensin II by an angiotensin-converting enzyme found in the lungs.

Angiotensin II causes the blood vessels to constrict, resulting in increased blood pressure. It also stimulates the adrenal cortex (the adrenals are triangular glands that sit on top of the kidneys). The aldosterone secreted by the adrenals results in the re-absorption of sodium and water by the kidneys into the blood. The resulting increase in blood volume also contributes to the increase in blood pressure. Hence, when the rennin-angiotensin-aldosterone system is over active it causes high blood pressure.

ACE inhibitors prevent the formation of angiotensin II. The angiotensin II receptor blockers impede the action of angiotensin II by preventing the binding of angiotensin II on the receptors of the blood vessels. The blood vessels therefore dilate, thus reducing the blood pressure.

ACE inhibitors are used to lower the blood pressure and fluid load allowing the heart to pump better and lessen the chances of heart failure. In addition they decrease the progression of kidney disease due to diabetes or high blood pressure.

8. Beta Blockers

Coronary artery disease results in the heart muscle complaining because of decreased blood flow and oxygen supply. The mainstay of coronary artery disease management is therefore to enhance the flow through the coronary arteries while reducing the oxygen demand of the heart.

The beta blockers act by the different mechanisms listed below:

- They reduce the oxygen requirement of the heart as they reduce the heart rate, thus the work of the heart is reduced as also the blood pressure.
- Increase the blood flow through the coronary arteries.
- Reduce the damage at the microvascular level.
- Allow more oxygen to be made available to the body tissues.
- Prevent aggregation of platelets.
- Protect the heart muscle.

The result is that the severity and frequency of angina is reduced. Beta-blockers are used in management of all types of coronary artery disease. They are started early in the treatment of an acute heart attack (myocardial treatment).

9. Calcium Channel Blockers

The beneficial effects of calcium channel blockers in the treatment of coronary artery disease are due to their:

- Ability to dilate the coronary arteries, which increases the blood flow to the heart muscle.
- Possible ability to prevent coronary artery spasms.
- Ability to lower the blood pressure which in turn reduces the workload on the heart.

- Allowing the heart muscles to use less oxygen and blood flow for their functioning.

- Ability to slow a fast heart rate and control irregular rhythms of the heart.

Studies suggest that calcium channel blockers also have plaque stabilization action. They help to lower the blood pressure in persons suffering from coronary artery disease. They are also used to help to relieve angina symptoms by reducing both the frequency and the severity of chest pain or discomfort.

10. Statins

Statins are among the most commonly prescribed drugs in patients with coronary artery disease. The statins have been shown to significantly reduce the risk of a heart attack and death in patients with proven coronary artery disease. In persons with high cholesterol levels who are at an increased risk for heart disease, they also reduce cardiac events. Although primarily recognized for their cholesterol lowering property the statins have several other beneficial effects, which can additionally improve the cardiac risk.

They are popularly known by the names atorvastatin, fluvastatin, lovastatin, simvastatin, rosuvastatin, pravastatin among others.

Primarily cholesterol-lowering drugs, statins act by inhibiting a liver enzyme which reduces the ability of the liver to produce cholesterol. They improve cholesterol levels by significantly reducing the 'bad' cholesterol levels (LDL), causing a small increase in the 'good' cholesterol levels (HDL) and moderately reducing triglyceride levels.

In addition to their effect in improving cholesterol levels, the other beneficial effects are their ability to reduce the plaque size in the arteries, they stabilize the plaques making plaque ruptures less likely, reducing the inflammation which triggers plaque formation, reduce the CRP levels and decrease the formation of blood clots. They are also supposed to improve overall vascular function.

11. Ezetimibe

Ezetimibe lowers the plasma cholesterol levels, by decreasing the absorption of cholesterol in the intestine. It can be used alone or in combination with statins, when statins alone are unable to control the cholesterol levels.

However, some clinical trials have shown that clinically significant outcomes like major coronary events did not improve and certain outcomes like thickening of the artery wall actually worsened. It is now suggested as a last resort drug.

12. Bile Acid Sequestrant

The body uses cholesterol to produce bile acids. Bile acid sequestrants prevent the body from reusing bile acids. The result is that the body must make more bile acids, using cholesterol to do so; as a result the blood LDL cholesterol levels are lowered. The bile acid sequestrants can also slightly increase the levels of the 'good' cholesterol. Cholestyramine and Colesevelam are examples of bile acid sequestrants. They can be used alone or in conjunction with statins.

13. Fibrates

Fibrates are drugs that lower the cholesterol. They primarily reduce the level of triglycerides in the blood, and also help to increase the levels of HDL cholesterol (good cholesterol) to a lesser degree. They also expel fats from the body and increase the amount of enzymes that break down fats in the blood.

Fibrates may be prescribed for heart-related conditions and often form part of the treatment plan. However, the use of fibrates remains controversial. Some studies suggest that they may be less beneficial in lowering cholesterol levels and reducing heart attacks and strokes, as compared to the other cholesterol lowering drugs.

14. Niacin

Vitamin B3, niacin or nicotinic acid helps in raising the levels of good cholesterol (HDL) by about 30% to 35%. It is considered as a secondary prevention therapy and is combined with other cholesterol lowering agents. A meta-analysis study has shown that niacin is associated with a significant reduction in cardiovascular events and a possible, small, non-significant decrease in mortality in coronary and cardiovascular diseases.

15. For the 'No Option' Group

Traditionally, for those suffering from severe angina, drug therapy, angioplasty or coronary artery bypass graft surgery is suggested as treatment modalities. There may still be a certain group of people, who despite undergoing these forms of treatment, experience-troubling chest pains. Some people may not be candidates for surgical intervention, angioplasty or stents, due to their age, additional heart problems or other health concerns.

Does this mean that there are no further options for these individuals and they have to continue to experience chest pain? There are some other forms of treatment, which are being studied and show promise. They are as follows.

- **Angiogenesis/Gene Therapy**

  An option currently under investigation involves 'angiogenesis', i.e., the formation of new blood-flow pathways. Use of gene therapy to trigger the creation or enlargement of blood vessels to the heart, thereby improving previously impaired blood flow is also under study.

- **Spinal Stimulation**

  Spinal stimulation involves the implantation of a small device that sends low-voltage electrical stimulation to the spinal cord to interrupt pain fibres. It is being studied as a way to block the sensation of chest pain. In patients with back and leg pain similar devices are used as a treatment option.

- **Transmyocardial Laser Revascularization**

  Transmyocardial Laser Revascularization (TMLR) is a surgical technique that uses lasers to create tiny channels. It is envisaged that these laser 'channels' could destroy nerve fibres that cause pain or stimulate the growth of new blood vessels.

  If left untreated, chronic angina can lead to an inactive lifestyle that may contribute to progression of the disease. New treatment techniques offer hope to patients who previously had few or no options for pain relief or treatment for their heart disease.

III. Time Is Crucial During a Heart Attack

During a heart attack time is of essence. About half the people who die of a heart attack will die before they reach the hospital. For every 30 minutes of decreased blood flow to the heart muscle there is an 8-10% increase in mortality.

Timely, efficient and appropriate therapy is the key to saving the heart muscle. It is best to receive treatment within the 'golden hour' i.e., within one hour after the symptoms start. This will improve the chances of survival and save the heart muscle.

It is therefore vital to first recognize the symptoms of a heart attack and then to get help at the earliest. This is true whether you are experiencing a heart attack yourself or are witness to someone else experiencing one.

The Warning Signs

Typically, there may be complaints of:
- A pain or squeezing sensation in the chest.
- Discomfort in one or both arms, back, neck, jaw and stomach.
- Shortness of breath or a feeling that it is difficult to breath.
- A cold sweat or profuse sweating.
- Nausea.
- A feeling of light-headedness or giddiness.

Out of these the most common complaints experienced are chest pain or chest discomfort. Certain signs and symptoms tend to occur together. Shortness of breath and chest pain may be associated with each other as may be sweating, nausea and neck pain.

A person might be unsure as to whether they are having a heart attack. This is probably because they expect the event to be dramatic—sudden chest pain and the person falls to the ground! The fact is that not all heart attacks are as sudden. Most people will experience symptoms that start slowly and get stronger gradually. At times the symptoms may wax and wane.

If Someone is Having a Heart Attack

If you suspect that someone is having a heart attack the most important thing to do is to call for professional help. Placing that call within the first three to five minutes should ensure treatment within the first hour, improving the chances for survival and limiting injury to the heart muscle.

Do not

- Leave the person alone except to call for help.
- Allow the person to deny the symptoms and convince you not to call for emergency help.
- Wait to see if the symptoms go away.
- Give the person anything by mouth except in the case that some form of heart medication (such as nitroglycerin) has been prescribed.
- Drive the person to the hospital yourself, unless there is no other choice. It wastes precious time and the driver cannot offer any help while driving.

In the ambulance, the emergency medical team is likely to have oxygen, pain-relieving medicines and equipment to monitor the patient. The paramedics are available to render care en route.

The advantage of calling for professional help/cardiac ambulance is that they may have facilities for an ECG which may detect a heart attack or a rhythm disturbance. The level of care needed can be decided and the patient taken to the appropriate centre to save time.

The emergency medical team might also have the following facilities:

- They may be in a position to offer medication that can bust the clot and halt the heart attack in progress.
- They would be equipped with a defibrillator that can be used to shock the heart back to a normal rhythm if needed.
- The patient can be moved to the hospital at the earliest.

71

- They will be in touch with the hospital, which can be alerted even before the patient reaches. When they reach the hospital, the individual can be treated faster.

If You Are Having a Heart Attack

- It is important to know the warning signs.
- Tell somebody if any warning signs are being experienced. If you are alone, decide whom to call and have their name and number handy. Share your health condition with your spouse, friend, colleague or doctor.
- Know when to call for medical help. If already under treatment the doctor would have instructed you when to call for help.
- Do not wait more than three to five minutes before calling for professional help especially if the symptoms are different or more severe than those in the past.

While Waiting for Help:

- Lie in a comfortable position.
- Loosen any tight clothing.
- Open a window if the room is unventilated.
- If already prescribed medication, follow the doctor's instructions.
- Minimize activity.

In an emergency, plan to go to the nearest hospital.

Cardiac Arrest

A heart attack could cause a cardiac arrest, where the heart stops beating and no blood is pumped to the body tissues and organs. Ten seconds into a cardiac arrest, a person loses consciousness. The patient becomes unresponsive. As the heart stops, the breathing may also stop completely i.e., the person is suffering a cardiopulmonary arrest. Without Cardio Pulmonary Resuscitation, or CPR, the patient dies.

Not all heart attacks lead to cardiac arrest. However, when it happens, professional help must be sought immediately and CPR started.

Nowadays, it is not uncommon to see special machines called Automated External Defibrillators (AEDs) that can shock the heart in cases of a cardiac arrest, stationed in public places like airports.

If available, the AED should be used before starting CPR or calling the EMS. They are very easy to use and it is suggested that one should learn how to use these machines.

IV. The Future for Coronary Artery Disease

"Hope is like a road in the country; there was never a road, but when many people walk on it, the road comes into existence."

— Lin Yutang

For better understanding of the disease process, early diagnosis and appropriate management, new tools, skills and techniques are being developed and learnt. While some are still in the experimental phase, others are already being used.

Understanding Genetic Susceptibility in CAD

The latest genetic techniques are being used to examine DNA from patients with heart disease to help identify the genes and molecules responsible for CAD. This is expected to help in the development of new diagnostic tools and treatment strategies.

It is anticipated that human genetics will not only help in predicting disease but also help to identify patients for whom specific pharmacologic or device-related treatments are optimal. This will help to develop specialized drugs for subpopulations.

New Horizons in Development and Use of Drugs

Given modern genetics and genomics and the identification of specific blood biomarkers that help differentiate patients with common disorders such as heart failure or atherosclerosis, greater targeted use of drugs is likely to emerge in the next decade or so. This will help to better tailor drugs for specific groups of patients and greatly improve therapeutic efficacy.

The concept of a 'polypill' refers to the inclusion of multiple drugs in a single tablet. This will allow a combination of several generic drugs in previously proven safe and effective dosages. It will be very useful in populations with limited resources and also improve compliance of medication.

Diagnostic Tools

- ### Optical Coherence Tomography

   Optical Coherence Tomography (OCT) is a new imaging technology. It helps in the diagnosis and treatment of cardiovascular disease. The system, consisting of a high-resolution camera and a light source, allows cardiologists to see inside the human heart arteries. It provides precise measurements of the dimensions of lesions as well as of the size and structure of the coronary artery. This allows the selection and placement of appropriate stents. The cardiologist is able to minimize the risk of the coronary vessels becoming narrow again and is able to guide follow-up treatment, using this information.

- ### Magnetic Resonance Imaging (MRI)

   The thickness of the coronary artery walls is a direct measurement of early-stage coronary artery disease. An MRI technique called time-resolved multi-frame acquisition uses five continuous images in order to increase the success rate of obtaining an image free of blurring.

   The technique allows one to detect any significant difference between the thickness of the walls of the arteries in coronary patients and those in healthy participants.

   The results suggest that MRI may be used in the future to screen for individuals at risk for coronary artery disease and could help to monitor the effects of therapies.

- ### Positron Emission Tomography (PET)

   PET is emerging as a powerful, non-invasive imaging tool for evaluating atherosclerosis in patients with known or suspected coronary artery disease. It has an edge over conventional Single-Photon Emission CT (SPECT) imaging in evaluating regional myocardial perfusion and metabolism in patients with CAD. PET scanners are now being converted to hybrid PET/CT devices. In the setting of CAD, they offer the potential of comprehensive non-invasive evaluation of the anatomy and function of the cardiac system.

Treatment Modalities

- **Nanotechnology**

  Nanoparticles are man-made structures engineered for specific uses. Their size is of the order of 10^{-9} to 10^{-7} m. Currently, stents are being used to widen narrowed vessels and deliver drugs. However, there are certain situations where a stent either cannot be used or may not be the treatment of choice.

  A nanotechnological treatment involves newly engineered nanoparticles, which bind to damaged vascular tissue and then release a drug that prevents the growth of thrombi around an atheroma. They are able to differentiate between healthy and damaged sections of the arterial endothelium.

  The treatment does not require surgery; the particles can be made up in solution, and administered intravenously. No additional procedures are needed.

- **Angiogenesis**

  If a person is diagnosed with a heart attack and there is damage to the heart muscle, then it is imperative that blood flow to the heart muscle be restored at the earliest. The possible conventional treatment options include:

  - Medicines.

  - Angioplasty to dilate the arteries where there are blockages, along with stenting, if required. Stents will act as scaffolding to prevent the artery from closing again, once it has been opened.

  - Coronary bypass surgery to create alternate channels to help the blood flow beyond the blocks.

  However, there is a new method of treatment, called angiogenesis, in which new blood vessels could be made to grow from the already existing ones. Although still in the experimental phase it offers new hope for the desperately ill.

  For many atherosclerotic diseases, like coronary heart disease, peripheral arterial disease and wound healing disorders, therapeutic angiogenesis clinical trials are being carried out worldwide, to provide a treatment option.

The three main categories of how the process of angiogenesis is stimulated are:

- **Gene Therapy**

  Some patients who suffer from blockages of the major coronary artery develop collateral arteries over time. These are smaller blood vessels that form alternate pathways for the blood to flow to compensate for the decreased blood flow in the main artery. Gene therapy is an attempt to duplicate the natural process. Its aim is to supply genetic material to the areas affected and thereafter allow the body to heal itself.

  Performed as a single catheterization lab procedure, it involves the injection of a virus carrying a gene that codes for a protein which promotes the growth of blood vessels.

- **Protein Therapy** (using angiogenic growth factors like FGF-1 or Vascular Endothelial Growth Factor (VEGF))

  There are certain factors that promote the growth of new blood vessels. The Fibroblast Growth Factor (FGF) and Vascular Endothelial Growth Factor (VEGF) are proteins that when injected into the heart have been equated to seeds from which new vessels will sprout. The result is the development of a network of new blood vessels.

  In the clinical trials that have been carried out so far, the proteins have been injected into the heart muscle during bypass surgery. Now, an improved technique using a needle tipped catheter introduced through a vessel in the leg is under consideration. It would be guided by X-Rays to decide the best site for injection. The protein factors would be delivered directly into the heart muscle from the inside.

- **Cell-based Therapies**

  Cell therapy is used as a way to treat damaged heart tissue. The patient's own adult stem cells are used. Permanent changes have been reported with this treatment. New blood vessels develop and the dead tissue in the heart is repaired.

  The patient is injected with a hormone, which causes the release of advantageous stem cells from their bone marrow into the bloodstream. The patient is then made to exercise on a treadmill. As a result of the physical exertion the stem cells travel quickly to their heart and start their action. They start creating new blood vessels helping to both restore the blood circulation and improve the overall function of the heart.

- **FGF9**

  It is suggested that the current methods used for angiogenesis as a treatment modality may not be successful because the new blood vessels formed do not last very long. They may not be able to actually control the flow of blood into the areas that need it. There is a need to 'support' the cells of the walls of the new vessels. Attempts are under way to use a protein called the Fibroblast Growth Factor 9 (FGF9) which would assist in 'supporting' the cells of new blood vessels as they are formed by the body.

  This new strategy will also ensure that smooth muscle cells surround the redeveloped vessels. This will allow them to relax and constrict ensuring that the right amount of blood and oxygen, reaches the tissues.

  Angiogenesis is obviously a natural process, so is there a way to stimulate it naturally? Angiogenesis is generally associated with aerobic and endurance exercise. The possibility of exercise helping to increase the blood vessel network in the heart is also under study.

Selected patient populations have benefited from the alternative therapy options. Having passed safety tests some are in the second phase of human trials. There are however, still some serious concerns that are being addressed, such as the following:

- With gene therapy there are risks of an immune response, potential toxicity, immunogenicity, inflammatory responses and oncogenesis related to the viral vectors. These considerations must be addressed seriously.

- The best way to deliver protein therapy still needs to be decided. If the protein is administered through oral, intra-arterial or intramuscular routes, it may not have the desired effect. The therapeutic protein could be metabolized or removed from the system before the target tissue is reached.

- The best cell types and the dosages to be used in cell therapy still need to be decided.

Angiogenesis therapy is a hope for patients suffering from atherosclerotic disorders.

Chapter 5

What is Different?

I. Heart Disease in Women

"Every time I close the door on reality it comes in through the windows."

— Jennifer Yane

Coronary artery disease has always been thought of as a 'man's' problem. It has been traditionally believed that the female hormones serve as coronary protection factors; that the female hormones protect women from coronary diseases from a young age until they reach menopause.

However, changing lifestyle habits seem to have levelled the gender advantage conferred by the female hormones. The fact is that in the United States, coronary artery disease is the number one cause of death in both men and women. In the United Kingdom coronary artery disease is the single largest cause of death in women, as is the case in most developed countries.

According to WHO statistics, the number of women suffering from coronary diseases has increased by 300% in the last five years.

Other types of heart disease like Coronary Microvascular Disease (CMD) and the broken heart syndrome also pose a threat to women.

The American Heart Association 2012 statistical fact sheet update on women & cardiovascular diseases reveals that:

- More than one in three female adults has some form of Cardiovascular Disease (CVD).
- About 7.5 million females today have CAD. Of these, 3.1 million have a history of Myocardial Infarction (MI, or a heart attack).
- Sixty four per cent of the women who died suddenly of CAD had no previous symptoms.

- 604,000 females diagnosed with CAD were discharged after a short-stay in hospital, in 2009.

Women fighting heart disease are not accurately diagnosed and do not receive the care they require when they need it. This has been attributed to the fact that women do not seek treatment as early as men do and also to the fact that they are not treated as aggressively.

Statistically, heart attacks are more deadly and disabling for women than they are for men. Twenty six per cent of women aged 45 and above who have an initial recognized MI (heart attack) die within a year, as compared to 19% of men.

The Plaque – Gender Difference

It appears that in women the hormonal or genetic differences change the way their arteries react, making them prone to this form of the disease. There may be a lesser propensity of women experiencing the traditional symptoms of crushing chest pain, difficulty in breathing and numbness in the left arm. Two-thirds of women experience none of these signs. The symptoms of a heart attack in women often tend to be subtle, frequently presenting as fatigue, sweating, nausea or jaw pain, which is probably the reason why they are often ignored.

In women the plaque along the walls of coronary arteries accumulates more diffusely being more evenly spread on vessel walls. Men tend to have bulges of plaque. The current diagnostic tests look for clumps of blockage making them less useful in women, which is probably why one-third of the women who have heart attacks show no blocks on these tests.

Does Gender Matter?

The statistics are scary and speak for themselves:

- Regardless of ethnicity or race, one in four women dies from CAD.
- While women today are more aware and understand that CAD is the number one cause of death in both men and women, they still do not associate their risk factors with a personal risk of developing CAD.

- Pre-hospital admission deaths from a heart attack are higher among women than men.

- Full recovery following a heart attack never occurs in two-thirds of women. Out of every three women one has some form of cardiovascular disease.

- Women with risk factors relating to ethnicity, obesity, a sedentary life, age more than 65, pre-diabetes or diabetes, high blood cholesterol or high blood pressure, carry a higher risk of developing CAD.

- Even the effectiveness of individual medical tests used to assess CAD show a gender variance.

- Use of birth control pills and hormone therapy which are specific to women are also said to carry a risk of CAD.

Over the last few decades the number of CAD related deaths in men has reduced significantly, which is not the case for women. The reasons for this discrepancy are possibly due to the fact that:

- Women tend to have more 'atypical' CAD related symptoms as compared to men.

- CAD is harder to detect in women since they have a greater chance of 'silent ischemia,' where the blood flow to the heart is restricted yet no chest pain is experienced.

- Men and women with the same degree of symptoms show different levels of obstructive CAD. The levels in women are much lower as compared to those in men. This is suggestive of a harder to detect, different disease pattern in women.

- Compared to men, women with obstructive CAD appear to have more adverse outcomes including a greater risk of dying.

It is important, given these differences that women learn to recognize their symptoms and get supportive and life-saving care at the earliest.

What is the Difference Due to

- **Low Index of Suspicion**

  The index of suspicion to detect CAD in women has always been low. For a long time, predominantly thought of a man's disease, CAD was often not considered when women complained. Considering the nature of work done by men their chest pain and heart attack were 'expected', while similar complaints in women were dismissed as non-specific or general malaise. They were expected to suffer only 'female problems'.

- **Microvascular Coronary Artery Disease**

  Research has shown that CAD in women can be more difficult to diagnose. Although, almost 50% of women have no apparent coronary artery blockage, they continue to suffer symptom-related disabilities. Until recently, they would have been dismissed and told that their symptoms were more in the mind, rather than physical.

  In a third of these women the cells of the endothelium (the lining of the inner surface of the arteries) malfunction, resulting in what is called microvascular coronary disease. This may be triggered by factors such as hypercholesterolemia, diabetes, high blood pressure, smoking and environmental factors.

In some women the cause of the chest pain and discomfort may relate to gall bladder disease, oesophageal reflux and other causes.

One Management Protocol Suits All

Once the fact that women can also suffer from CAD was accepted, it was presumed that the same treatment and protocols would work equally effectively in both genders. What was overlooked was that all the drug trials till almost the mid 1990s, were exclusively conducted in males; even older women were excluded.

Also, the therapy offered to women often tended to be inferior and less aggressive as compared to that given to men. The early 21st century saw research becoming more unbiased. Women were being objectively included in health and medical-related research; which clearly showed that the recommended treatments tended to be underused and delayed in women be it beta blockers, early aspirin, reperfusion treatment or an emergency angioplasty.

Considering that CAD remains the leading cause of death in both genders worldwide, serious attention needs to be paid to the preventive and treatment aspects of care.

Irrespective of ethnicity or age there is a need for women to be aware of the risk factors as also the possible signs and symptoms of both CAD and heart attack.

Risk Factors

While both the modifiable and non modifiable risk factors are similar in both genders, certain subtle differences do exist.

- Women tend to have smaller coronary arteries. There is a hormonal bias.

- **Age:** Between the ages of 45 and 65, CAD kills more women than breast cancer. By the age of 60 women are as likely as men to suffer from a heart attack.

- **Family history:** If a sibling or one parent has died before the age of 55, because of CAD, the risk increases.

- **Body size:** If the weight is 30% above the ideal body weight, particularly if fat collects around the waist rather than the buttocks or hips, the risk increases.

- **Unhealthy lipid profile:** High total cholesterol (over 200), low HDL (under 45) high triglycerides (over 200) and high LDL, or 'bad' cholesterol (over 130) increase the risk of CAD.

- **High blood pressure:** Hypertensive women (those whose blood pressure is over 150/90) have an increased risk for stroke, kidney and heart disease. As women age, their chances of developing high blood pressure are greater than those for men.

- **Diabetes:** A survey conducted by Metropolis Healthcare over a period of six months, from April to September 2010, showed that in 2010, one million more women than men had diabetes (143 million women as against 142 million men). The difference is expected to increase to six million by 2030 (222 million women against 216 million men). Diabetes increases women's risk for CAD four-to-six fold.

- **Menopause:** Premature menopause (before the age of 38) increases the risk for CAD. Natural menopause is not a disease. But taking Hormonal Replacement Therapy (HRT) may help keep good cholesterol (HDL) levels high if they are too low (below 45 for women).

Lifestyle Related Risk Factors

- **Smoking:** It remains the single most important risk factor that escalates the chances of CAD. Among Americans aged 18 years or more, 20.4 million women (17.5%) are smokers. Younger women are now taking to smoking. Women who smoke risk having a heart attack 19 years earlier than women who do not smoke.

- **Sedentary lifestyle:** Lack of physical exercise increases the risk of CAD. In 2010, only 16.4% of women aged 18 and above met the requirements of the 2008 Federal Physical Activity Guidelines.

- **Stress:** More and more women are leaving the comfort of the four walls of their homes, and taking on more responsibilities as part of the work force. They juggle home and office responsibilities; and play multiple roles as daughter, mother, wife, daughter-in-law, office employee, etc. The combination of many responsibilities, a lot of which are troublesome and unrewarding can lead to stress that increases the risk of CAD.

- **Birth control pills:** Oral contraceptives can increase the risk of CAD. In some women, oral contraceptives can lead to high blood pressure, another risk factor for CAD.

- **Substance abuse:** Cocaine can give even teenagers a fatal heart attack.

The National Institutes of Health launched the *Women's Ischemia Syndrome Evaluation* (WISE). It has been tracking about 1,000 women who have had pain or other symptoms, but seem fine on standard tests, since 1996. The aim is to document that heart disease is a fundamentally different disease in women in many ways which needs to be taken into consideration. The WISE study showed that many women whose arteries looked clear in angiograms and other standard tests had a significantly elevated risk of having a heart attack or dying within four or five years! When the researchers used ultrasound and other more sophisticated techniques to examine their arteries, they found that many actually had abnormalities. The women also scored higher on certain tests, such as those measuring levels of inflammation.

The Hormonal Bias

Estrogen the female hormone secreted by women during their reproductive years is considered cardio protective when the ovaries produce it naturally. The ovarian hormones, cause women to have, on an average, lower blood pressure than men until menopause. Hormonal differences also play a protective role in lowering blood cholesterol in younger women. However, after menopause, higher blood cholesterol makes women more susceptible to blocked coronary arteries, particularly in the presence of high triglycerides, another fatty substance that circulates in the blood. Whether the female hormones offer the same benefit when introduced artificially is controversial.

Many women might also take some form of hormones at some point in their life, such as:

- **Birth control pills:** Birth control or oral contraceptive pills may not increase the risk of coronary artery disease in healthy, young women who do not smoke, but can increase the risk in woman with other significant risk factors for CAD. Birth control pills may raise the level of the 'bad' cholesterol (LDL) and lower levels of the 'good' cholesterol (HDL).

- **Hormone therapy:** While natural hormones are protective in women, for those in the menopausal or postmenopausal period taking oestrogen alone or in combination with progestin will not prevent coronary artery disease. Taking hormonal therapy ten or more years after menopause may in fact raise the risk of coronary artery disease.

Otherwise healthy women under 35 years of age, who use oestrogen-based oral contraceptive pills or patches to practice birth control, are not considered at an increased risk of developing CAD. However, health issues like high blood pressure are associated with women over 35 years of age who are taking birth control pills or using patches. In postmenopausal women, the ovarian supply of hormones dips resulting in the typical postmenopausal symptoms like hot flushes, osteoporosis and a rise in certain cancers. In a bid to treat these problems and protect women, an attempt was made to replace the hormones using Hormone Replacement Therapy (HRT) or Postmenopausal Hormone Therapy (PHT). The effects and side effects of various hormonal preparations with only oestrogen or a combination of oestrogen and progestin were studied. These studies indicated that the therapy should be targeted and specific.

Signs and Symptoms

Given that the basic changes and pattern of involvement of the coronary arteries is different in women, it follows that the way they experience chest pain or heart attack may differ. While some may experience typical chest pain, tingling typically down the left arm, profuse sweating, shortness of breath and giddiness, others may experience less specific symptoms, such as pain in the neck, jaw, back or stomach, indigestion, nausea, vomiting, shortness of breath, heartburn, coughing, loss of appetite, or heart flutters. Sometimes chest pain may present as fatigue, anxiety or even insomnia.

The intensity of the symptoms tends to increase over time.

Since women tend to have heart attacks later in life than men, they may often suffer from other diseases (such as arthritis or osteoporosis) that can mask the symptoms of a heart attack.

It is important that women understand the signs and symptoms of CAD and heart attack, so that they can recognize them and seek timely help.

Identifying the Problem

The exercise stress test, or stress ECG, may be less accurate in women. Certain studies have shown that the Dobutamine stress echocardiography and exercise thallium myocardial scintigraphy are more reliable methods of diagnosing coronary artery disease in women.

An angiography can be used to identify CAD although microvascular disease is hard to detect.

Treatment

Women tend to 'sit on their problems' longer before seeking help. Also a higher index of suspicion is needed to pick up those with potential cardiac issues. Whether a medical or surgical line of management is intended, the important thing is early recognition and institution of the appropriate therapy.

Prevention

Women are central to their families. They are the pivots; controllers of promoting and maintaining healthy eating habits, a healthy lifestyle, and ensuring regular medication of any health issues. Women are often role models; when women make heart healthy lifestyle choices, their families often do too.

Aspirin

Aspirin is considered as a 'wonder drug' and a daily, low dose of aspirin has been promoted as a way of reducing the risk of CAD in men.

Surprisingly, it is only in women above 65 years and older that aspirin provides consistent benefits and significantly reduces the risk of a heart attack. In younger women it has been shown that aspirin does not seem to significantly reduce the risk of a heart attack, but it can reduce a first stroke by 20%. This can probably be explained by the nature of plaques seen in men and women. This gender difference may be related to the way men and women accumulate plaque in small arteries (which can lead to a stroke) and larger arteries (which can lead to a heart attack) or how they metabolize aspirin.

This difference is only relevant when aspirin is being used to prevent a first heart attack. In both men and women who had already suffered a heart attack, a daily low dose of aspirin was of equal benefit in preventing recurrent attacks.

Make Those Changes

It is necessary for all persons diagnosed with CAD to understand and address the modifiable risk factors that increase the chances of a heart attack.

Some principles that should be followed are:

- Eat right, sleep right, exercise right.
- Stop smoking.
- Control lipid levels in the blood, control blood pressure and control blood sugars.
- Understand and take the medicines as prescribed.
- Get regular medical check-ups.
- Do not ignore warning signs.
- Get advice before taking any hormonal treatments.
- Get into a cardiac rehabilitation programme to boost physical strength and increase endurance.

The Broken Heart Syndrome (Stress-Induced Cardiomyopathy/Takotsubo Cardiomyopathy)

As compared to men women are more likely to have a condition called the broken heart syndrome. Recently recognized, it is suggested that extreme emotional stress can lead to severe, albeit short-term, heart muscle failure. It can mimic a heart attack and may be misdiagnosed as such. Being essentially a heart muscle failure there is no suggestion of the coronary arteries being blocked. Most people would recover quickly and completely.

The hearts of women are vulnerable to developing irregular beats; the changing oestrogen (female hormone) levels are said to increase the sensitivity to irregular heartbeats and palpitations. Testosterone, the male hormone, has a protective effect.

In any case it is important to know your risks; know the signs and symptoms and seek timely help.

II. Children and Coronary Artery Disease

"A patient was admitted with a feeling of congestion in the chest. With reluctance she was referred to a cardiologist. The ECG showed extensive damage to the heart muscle and a coronary angiography showed 100% blockages in the major coronary arteries. A coronary angioplasty and stenting were carried out," said Dr B K Goyal,

Chief Cardiologist, Bombay Hospital. He continued after a pause, "The girl was nine years old."

Coronary artery disease has long been considered a disease of the elderly. India a country struggling with problems of malnutrition, also paradoxically has the tenth largest overweight population in the world, with children accounting for a significant number.

An Indian study conducted in a Delhi school has shown a strong positive correlation between the birth weights of children and their subsequent growth performance. It was concluded that the percentage of obese/overweight children and adolescents belonging to the upper strata of society is on the increase. A few years ahead this will translate into a group of overweight individuals, in the prime of their life, who are prone to a number of diseases including heart disease.

Today, 'younger' individuals are being diagnosed with coronary artery disease. Studies suggest that chronic diseases are biologically programmed right from the time one is in the womb. Dr Bhupendra Avasthi, Chief of the Pediatric Department at Lilavati Hospital and Surya Children's Hospital, Santa Cruz, says, "In the case of heart disease, it is hypothesized that under nutrition of the baby during middle gestation, increases the risk of later disease by the programming of blood pressure, cholesterol metabolism, blood coagulation and hormonal settings."

Dr Avasthi adds, "In addition, teenagers start making individual choices and developing personal lifestyles during adolescence. Many of these lifestyle choices such as diet patterns, the development of obesity, physical activity, cigarette smoking, and the use of oral contraceptives increase their risk factors for coronary artery disease."

Compelling evidence proves that fatty deposits or their forerunner begin in childhood and progress slowly into adulthood. The data from the Vietnam wartime autopsies confirms the presence of mature plaques by the end of the second decade of life! Therefore the importance of preventing this build up in the first and second decade of life cannot be stressed enough.

Risk Factors

Considering that the behaviour patterns of children parallel those of their parents the risk factors are also similar: family history, high levels of cholesterol, hypertension, smoking, diabetes, obesity, and physical inactivity. Hypothyroidism, environmental factors and economic factors may also contribute to the risk.

- **Hypercholesterolemia:** Elevated blood cholesterol is documented as one of the major causes of coronary artery disease. A family history of hyperlipoproteinemia and the type of fats consumed in the diet are said to influence serum lipid levels, and subsequently affect development of fatty deposits in the blood vessels.

  Since, when one should start cholesterol testing in childhood, and the cut-off point for hypercholesterolemia in teenagers still remain unclear, all adolescents must be screened to accurately identify those with hypercholesterolemia.

- **Hypertension:** The role of hypertension as a risk factor is clear. Those who have a family history of high blood pressure as well as children suffering from hypertension are likely to be hypertensive adults. This increases the risk of early coronary artery disease. In a study of healthy school-going children from northern India between the ages of 5 and 14 years, the prevalence of hypertension was found to be 11.7 per cent. Excessive salt intake and obesity also contribute to the development of hypertension.

- **Smoking:** The incidence of coronary artery disease and hypertension is higher in those who begin smoking before the age of 20.

- **Diet:** Childrens' food habits gravitate towards fast foods. Pizzas, French fries, chips, burgers and fizzy drinks are at the top of the list. These foods are loaded with salt, preservatives, trans fats and calories and predispose towards hypertension, obesity and coronary artery disease.

- **Obesity:** Obesity is associated with high blood pressure and abnormalities of serum lipids and carbohydrate metabolism. The first one to two years of life are the only times fat cells can multiply. It thus appears that early infancy may be the most important period for weight control on a permanent basis.

- **Physical activity:** Moderate physical activity is important for the normal growth and development of children. The activities of the younger generation are centred around computer games, the internet and television. Everything is remote controlled. Physical activity has taken a back seat. This further contributes to obesity and coronary artery disease.

Early appropriate intervention has the potential for a life time of effectiveness. Based on available data it is important that:

- Proper maternal nutrition should be instituted and maintained during pregnancy.
- Mother's milk, which is low in sodium content, is the best food for all infants. Breast feeding should be encouraged.
- A healthy lifestyle should be encouraged for all children.
- Children should be encouraged to start and maintain a regular daily exercise program under parental supervision.
- Cigarette smoking should be discouraged.
- Regular aerobic exercise that lasts at least 30–60 minutes on most days of the week should be encouraged.
- High blood pressure should be identified and treated.
- Obesity should be avoided or reduced.
- Diabetes mellitus should be diagnosed and treated.

Children aged two years and older should be encouraged to eat at least five servings of fruits and vegetables daily as well as a wide variety of other foods low in saturated fats and cholesterol.

Discourage:
- Overeating.
- The consumption of salted snacks.
- The intake of foods rich in cholesterol, saturated fats and sodium.

This will help children maintain normal blood cholesterol levels and promote cardiovascular health.

Modifying the risk factors for coronary artery disease at an early age, can prevent or at least delay the disease process.

III. Thyroid and Heart Disease

A small butterfly shaped organ located in the lower neck, the thyroid, orchestrates many vital body functions (Fig. 14). The hormones produced by it affect the functioning of almost all the body organs including the heart. It actually tells the body cells how much energy to use.

The thyroid hormones are important for normal cardiac function. Disorders of the thyroid have the potential to worsen old cardiac symptoms, cause new ones or speed up underlying heart problems.

The thyroid has to be thought of whenever cardiac symptoms worsen.

Thyroid disorders can lead to insufficient hormone production (hypothyroidism) or excess hormone production (hyperthyroidism).

Hypothyroidism

Hypothyroidism is more commonly associated with heart problems. Insufficient hormone production can slow the heart rate and affect the heart's functions. Hypothyroidism has the propensity to weaken the heart muscle and affect its pumping capacity.

Typical cardiac symptoms of hypothyroidism are:

- Shortness of breath on physical exertion and a poor exercise tolerance. This indicates worsening heart failure in patients with heart disease.
- A heart rate that is typically ten to twenty beats slower per minute than normal.
- An increased tendency to develop irregular heart rhythms in persons having an underlying heart problem.
- High blood pressure, as hypothyroidism tends to make the arteries stiffer causing the blood pressure to rise.
- Heart failure, or in those already suffering from a heart problem it can aggravate the problem.

- Swelling due to heart failure as well as swelling known as myxoedema due to accumulation of abnormal proteins and other molecules.
- An increase in the levels of bad cholesterol and the C-reactive proteins, which can hasten the underlying coronary artery disease.

In women, hypothyroidism is very common, yet it gets diagnosed late. Neither the individual nor the family considers weight gain or slowing down in activities among women to be alarming. A treatable condition, if left undiagnosed, it can cause damage to the heart functions. A common cause of hypothyroidism is a low intake of iodine, which is easily preventable.

Hyperthyroidism

Hyperthyroidism causes the heart muscle to work faster. In those suffering from hyperthyroidism there is an unexplained increase in heart rate. It may be associated with hypertension and the heart muscle is overworked.

The typical cardiac symptoms of hyperthyroidism are:

- Even on mild exertion the heart rate increases disproportionately. There is an increased tendency to develop fast, irregular, heart rhythms.
- Raised blood pressure due to the increased force of heart contractions.
- Shortness of breath, either due to a worsening heart failure or due to weakness of the skeletal muscles.
- Rarely hyperthyroidism can cause heart failure. If an individual already has a pre-existing heart problem it can worsen it.
- Worsening angina. Persons suffering from pre-existing coronary heart disease may experience an increase in chest pain or even a heart attack.

If a person is eating well but still losing weight then hyperthyroidism should be suspected.

If a thyroid problem is suspected during an examination of a patient with coronary artery disease, then thyroid investigations, which can include imaging and blood tests to check the values of the T3, T4 and TSH levels, are advised.

The American Thyroid Association in fact recommends routine screening for thyroid dysfunction in all individuals every five years from the age of 35 years onwards.

Undetected under or over functioning of the thyroid can cause harm to the heart. Once the thyroid problem is diagnosed and treatment initiated the associated heart problems can also be better controlled.

Chapter 6

The Body, Diet and Weight Control

I. Understanding Your Body

We live in an era of fast cars, colas, burgers, computers and remote controls. Lifestyle related diseases are the price one pays for economic prosperity and the modern way of life. No doubt the genetic make-up of a person contributes to the risk of heart disease, but it is one's lifestyle that becomes the deciding factor.

Regular consumption of foods high in calories and fats, soft drinks and desserts contribute to the increasing number on the weighing scale. A sedentary lifestyle, increasing age, certain hormonal disturbances and medications are all potential reasons for weight gain. Certain women find it difficult to lose the weight gained during pregnancy. Some people eat when they are depressed as they find it comforting, and tend to overeat especially the wrong kinds of foods.

A good saying to remember is, "A moment on the lips is a lifetime on the hips."

No doubt fat is vital for certain functions in the body, but while some extra fat can be carried by the body, after a certain point, it interferes with health. Being overweight puts one at risk for numerous health problems, such as:

- High blood pressure.
- Type 2 diabetes.
- Abnormal blood fats.
- Coronary artery disease.
- Stroke.
- Osteoarthritis, most often affecting the knees, hips and lower back. Excess weight puts extra pressure on these joints. This causes the cartilage protecting them to wear out, resulting in joint pain and stiffness.

- Gout, a disorder of the joints.

- Sleep apnoea, which is a serious condition. It causes a person to stop breathing for short periods when they are asleep and to snore heavily.

- Cancers associated with being overweight in women include those of the breast, uterus, cervix, ovaries and gall bladder. While overweight men have a particularly higher risk of cancers of the colon, rectum and the prostate.

- Fatty liver disease caused by fatty accumulation in the liver can cause cirrhosis of the liver.

- Gall bladder disease can be caused by deposition of excess cholesterol in the gall bladder. The risk of gallstones is higher in obese people. Rapid weight loss, due to strict or fad diets, of more than 2-3 kgs a week can also increase the risk of gallstones.

- Being overweight also has social implications and overweight people are often made fun of, which can result in depression, anger and mood swings.

Even modest amounts of weight loss, lower blood pressure, reduce the risk of cardiovascular disease and stroke, improve glucose control in diabetes, lower the chances of osteoarthritis and sleep apnoea as also the risk of cancer. The first goal in dealing with obesity is to achieve and maintain a healthier weight.

Certain guidelines help to decide whether one is entering the danger zone. They are as follows:

Body Mass Index (BMI)

The BMI is a formula that uses weight and height to estimate body fat and health risks. BMI is a measure of how healthy your weight is for your height. A BMI between 19 and 24 is considered a healthy weight range for a given height; between 25 and 29 is overweight and 30 or greater more is categorized as obese.

Waist Circumference

The body stores any spare fat under the skin as well as around vital organs in the abdomen. The fat stored in the abdomen is more problematic compared to the fat on the thighs or the buttocks.

If the amount of fat around the tummy is more the chances of developing type 2 diabetes and heart disease increase.

To find your correct waist size, feel your hip bone on one side. Then move your hand upwards until you feel the bones of your bottom rib. Between the two lies the waist, which may coincide with your navel.

To know your shape calculate the waist-to-hip ratio:

1. Measure your waist.
2. Measure your hips.
3. Divide the measurement of your waist by the measurement of your hips.

A waist to hip ratio of 0.85 or more in women or 1.0 or more in men suggests excess weight around the middle.

Depending on the distribution of fat in your body, your shape is defined. If you carry excess weight around your abdomen, that means you have an 'apple' shape. Those who carry excess fat around the buttocks and thighs are said to be 'pear' shaped.

- **Apple shaped:** Most of the fat is around the waist or upper body. This suggests that there is more fat deposited around the abdominal organs. Abdominal fat increases the risk of many of the serious conditions associated with obesity.
- **Pear shaped:** Most of the fat is around the hips and thighs or lower body. This is the preferred shape.

A woman's waist should measure less than 90 cms, while a man's waist measurement should be less than 100 cms.

Only when the risks are understood and it is realized that there is a need to act, can corrective steps be taken. It is necessary to understand one's body to be able to determine which foods and exercise will serve the purpose the best.

The mantra to a healthy weight and body remains 'eating right and burning more calories than you are eating'. However, it is not uncommon for the same diet and exercise plan to result in different outcomes in different people. It is necessary that the diet and exercise plan be tailored to suit individual requirements.

In his book titled *Atlas of Men* published in 1954, Shaldon described three body 'somatotypes'. It was suggested that the mental characteristics of an individual could be determined form the body type. The somatotypes described were:

- **Ectomorphic:** Characterized by long, thin muscles/limbs and also low fat storage. What we traditionally refer to as slim. They are the lucky ones who do not have a tendency to either store fat or build muscle.
- **Mesomorphic:** Characterized by a solid torso, medium bones, a narrow waist, wide shoulders and also low levels of fat. They are the ones we typically refer to as being muscular.
- **Endomorphic:** Characterized by increased fat storage, a large bony structure and a wide waist. What is referred to as fat. They have a tendency towards fat storage.

All others would be various combinations of the above three types.

Depending on the body type it was suggested that:

An ectomorphic person should train hard but in a controlled manner and under supervision, as he/she is not basically an athlete and there is a tendency to over train. Frequent, two hourly meals at least six times a day are advised to ensure enough nutrients for the body. It is generally advised that the calories obtained from proteins, carbohydrates and fats should be in the ratio 40:40:20.

A person who is endomorphic has to concentrate on losing fat. More cardio exercises are recommended for this group. It is suggested that they eat at least six meals a day, drink plenty of water and cut down on carbohydrates. The carbohydrates consumed should be such that they are slowly absorbed. More proteins should be eaten to get the required amounts of essential fatty acids.

Mesomorphic persons only need to practice moderation. They need to have exercise regimes, frequent meals, drink plenty of water, eat slowly and maintain a caloric ratio from proteins, carbohydrates and fats of 40:40:20.

One should always eat slowly to ensure proper absorption of the nutrients and avoid over eating.

A healthy diet, exercise and change in lifestyle can lead to a loss or gain in weight as desired. Only the morbidly obese need more drastic measures. Weight loss or gain under medical supervision is advised.

II. Diet and Weight Control

The importance of correct diet and nutrition cannot be stressed enough. At the end of the day what is needed is a healthy balanced, 'right' diet. Understanding the body type and the three main types of nutrients – carbohydrates, proteins and fats – will help the formulation of a realistic diet, which can be ratified by the dietician.

Carbohydrates

Foods rich in carbohydrates contain the most sugars (glucose) and are an almost instant source of energy. Each gram of carbohydrate gives 4 calories of energy. The body converts 100% of the carbohydrate containing foods into glucose and the extra glucose is stored in the liver as glycogen. Once the liver stores are full the extra carbohydrates are converted into fat.

The Glycemic Index or Glycaemic Index (GI) measures how fast your blood sugar level rises after eating a particular type of food. This is important. It is well documented that the damage to the body tissues happens because of sudden glucose spikes and dips. What is needed is a steady level of glucose in the blood.

Foods with carbohydrates that break down quickly during digestion, resulting in a rapid release of glucose into the blood have a high GI; whereas foods with carbohydrates that break down more slowly, releasing glucose more gradually into the bloodstream, tend to have a low GI.

Foods are classified as having a low, medium or high GI.

- Foods with low GI, 55 or less: e.g., some beans like soya beans white and black kidney beans; walnuts, peanuts; flax seeds, pumpkin seeds, sesame seeds; lentils; grains like wheat, millet, oat, rye, barley; fruits like peaches and strawberries and almost all vegetables.

- Foods with a medium GI of 56 to 69: e.g., grape juice, raisins, bananas, pita bread, Basmati rice, prunes.

- Foods with a high GI of 70 or more: e.g., white bread, potatoes, most varieties of white rice, cornflakes, glucose, pretzels.

Foods with a high GI, like glucose which has a GI of 100 will cause a sudden spike in the blood glucose level. This is particularly important for diabetic patients where a lower glycaemic response, mostly but not always, equates to a lower demand of insulin, and may help to improve long-term control of blood glucose and blood lipids.

The glycaemic index does not however account for the quantity of carbohydrates consumed. This is taken into account by the glycaemic load which is determined by multiplying the carbohydrate content of the actual serving by the glycaemic index.

Using the above concept carbohydrates are classified as:

- **Healthy carbohydrates:** Also called complex or slower-acting carbohydrates, they include multigrain bread, brown rice, lentils and beans. This type of carbohydrate raises blood sugar slowly and the effect lasts longer. This helps to keep you from feeling hungry for a longer time and to keep blood sugar levels closer to normal.

- **Not-so-healthy carbohydrates:** Also known as simple or fast-acting carbohydrates, they include candy, cookies, cake, soda, juice and sweetened beverages. This type of carbohydrate raises blood sugar levels very quickly, but the effect does not last very long. This is the reason why these carbohydrates work well to correct low-blood sugar but do not satisfy hunger as well as the healthy carbohydrates do.

Proteins

Proteins give 4 calories per gram. In a healthy diet, proteins constitute approximately 12-20% of the total daily caloric intake.

Proteins are the body building blocks. They are needed for repair, growth, maintenance and energy. They can also be stored and are used mainly by the muscles. Sixty per cent of the proteins are converted into glucose by the body.

Proteins release glucose slowly over three to four hours. Foods with a high protein content do not cause the blood sugar level to rise too much.

Fats

Of all the nutrients fats contribute the maximum number of calories - 9 calories per gram. In a healthy diet, about 30% of the total daily calories should come from fats. Fats also contribute to the body's energy, but only about 10% of the fat is converted into glucose by the body.

Although fat per se does not impact the blood sugar much, when fat is consumed with carbohydrates it slows the rise of blood sugar. Fats however slow down digestion and once the blood sugar has risen it tends to stay higher for a longer time.

There are constant advisory notices about eating unsaturated fats, avoiding trans fats and saturated fats. So what exactly are these fats?

Fats in the Food

- **Saturated fats** are derived from animal products like eggs, meat and dairy products; palm, palm kernel and coconut oil. Saturated fats tend to be solid at room temperature. They raise both the total and LDL cholesterol levels. While the earlier dictum was to avoid them totally, there is now a school of thought that suggests that there are different kinds of saturated fats that may have a more neutral effect on cholesterol.

- **Unsaturated fats** are derived from plant and vegetable sources. Monounsaturated fats and polyunsaturated fats are two types of unsaturated fatty acids; both are liquid at room temperature.

- **Monounsaturated Fats (MUFAs):** While liquid at room temperature, they start to solidify at cold temperatures. This type of fat is found in canola oil, olives, olive oil, nuts, avocados and peanut oil and is preferable to other fats. Studies have shown MUFAs can actually lower LDL cholesterol and maintain HDL cholesterol.

- **Polyunsaturated Fats (PUFAs):** These are found in sesame, corn, safflower and soyabean oils and cottonseed and have also been shown to reduce LDL cholesterol levels. However, too much can also lower the HDL cholesterol.

- **Hydrogenated or trans fats** are actually unsaturated fats used to extend the shelf life of processed foods like cakes, chips and cookies. They can raise both the total and LDL cholesterol levels while also lowering HDL cholesterol levels. These are best avoided.

- **Omega-3 fatty acids** include an 'essential' fatty acid that is crucial for health but is not manufactured by our bodies. Cold-water fish, flax seeds, soya and walnuts are good sources of omega-3 fatty acids. These reduce the risk of coronary heart disease and also boost the immune system.

One should choose mono unsaturated or poly-unsaturated fats, limit saturated and trans fats and consume sufficient quantities of essential fatty acids.

Weight Loss

There are certain medications that are available to help one lose weight. The common prescription medicines either block the absorption of some fats (e.g., Orlistat) or create a feeling of fullness (e.g., Sibutramine). They are not meant for people who want to lose a few pounds for cosmetic reasons, but for obese persons, and should always be taken under medical supervision. Some of the over-the-counter supplements promising to help burn fat faster or reduce hunger may have dangerous side effects. A healthy diet along with exercise is the best way to lose weight. A vitamin supplement may help to close the nutritional gap.

Behavioural Strategies

These are techniques for initiating and maintaining changes in lifestyle that may result in sustained weight loss. A counsellor may be helpful. Certain obese people suffer from eating disorders and may require psychotherapy. It is important to treat the eating disorder before an obese person attempts to lose weight.

Surgery for Weight Loss

When all serious efforts to lose weight, including diet and exercise fail, surgery may be indicated. This decision requires a pre-operative evaluation by a surgeon, endocrinologist, dietician and psychologist. Certain selection criteria decide which patients need surgical intervention.

A medical evaluation is carried out. The investigations required are routine haematology and biochemistry studies; vitamin, iron and calcium studies; hormonal studies; an ultrasound or CT scan of the abdomen; a genomic study (Leptin or OB gene); pulmonary function tests in the case of sleep apnoea and a cardiac evaluation.

Various surgical options are available. Of these liposuction is a cosmetic surgery, and is not intended for weight loss.

Bariatric surgery aims to reduce the capacity of the stomach by using a band or staples. It helps patients who eat large amounts of food. After the operation, the patient is only able to eat small quantities and yet feels satisfied.

Bariatric surgery plus intestinal bypass techniques are intended for those who eat rich, oily and sugary foods. They reduce the quantity that one can eat while also reducing the calories absorbed by the body.

One should avoid reaching a stage where one needs surgery. It is advisable keep your weight under check. Weight loss is a long battle and needs perseverance.

III. Heart Healthy: Alternate Therapies, Foods and Supplements

One often reads in the papers that one should eat fish regularly, and take Omega-3 and Vitamin C tablets as this will help to protect your heart. There are some supplements and alternative therapies that have been suggested as ways of controlling risk factors, e.g., lowering triglyceride levels, lowering LDL levels, raising HDL levels, controlling diabetes, hypertension and atherosclerosis, controlling weight and obesity and even preventing plaque formation. Some are proven, while some are still under investigation, and others have definitely been discounted.

Like any medicine, anything with an effect is likely to have a side effect. Alternate therapies, foods or supplements may have inherent side effects or interact adversely with the medicine that has been advised by your doctor, so if you are taking or experimenting with any alternate medicines or therapies, it should be in consultation with your doctor.

Foods and Supplements

- ### Fish Oils

  The American Heart Association says that the Omega-3 fatty acids contained in fish oils can improve the heart health of normal individuals, people at risk for cardiovascular disease and people living with cardiovascular disease. Omega-3 fatty acids reduce triglyceride levels, slowing build up of plaque and help to reduce blood pressure. They also reduce the risk of abnormal heartbeats or arrhythmias, which can lead to sudden death. Consumption of fatty fish is advised at least twice a week. Omega-3 fatty acids are also available in capsule form and can be taken under medical advice.

- ### Garlic

  Garlic, a culinary herb, is widely used for the treatment and prevention of cancer and cardiovascular disease. It is suggested that garlic may reduce total cholesterol and triglyceride levels.

- ### Artichoke Extract

  Artichokes a spiny vegetable, contain a compound called cynarin, which increases the production of bile by the liver while also boosting bile flow from the gall bladder. Bile is integral to the excretion of excess cholesterol from the body, which helps to increase the levels of 'good cholesterol' while reducing levels of the 'bad cholesterol'.

- ### Barley

  Barley is a whole grain which contains vitamins and antioxidants and beta-glucan an important soluble fibre, which aids in lowering blood cholesterol levels. It reduces the absorption of cholesterol and fat into the bloodstream. Barley is said to improve digestive health, aid improvement of blood glucose levels in diabetics and help heart health by lowering the triglyceride levels and the LDL levels while boosting HDL levels.

- ### Beta-sitosterol

  Beta-sitosterol is a plant sterol, found in rice bran, wheat germ, corn oil and soybeans. It has a chemical structure similar to that of cholesterol. It is suggested for benign prostatic hypertrophy, lowering cholesterol, increasing immunity and reducing inflammation.

- **Coenzyme Q10**

  Coenzyme Q10 or CoQ10 produced by the body is needed for cellular function. In most people CoQ10 levels fall with age. In people with certain medical conditions such as heart disease, cancer, muscular dystrophy, diabetes and Parkinson's disease, the levels of CoQ10 are found to be low.

  Although, the beneficial effects of CoQ10 in heart disease and other conditions remain controversial, in those suffering from coronary artery disease it may reduce angina and improve exercise tolerance. More research is still needed to confirm its efficacy for the prevention or treatment of coronary heart disease.

- **Vitamin C**

  Increased consumption of Vitamin C may help to prevent coronary artery disease. Vitamin C deficiency is said to play an integral role in heart attack and stroke. Vitamin C boosts the production of elastin and collagen molecules that support the blood vessels. Vitamin C therapy could help prevent coronary artery disease by repairing blocked arteries and other damage to the blood vessels. This would significantly reduce the risk of heart attack and stroke.

- **Plant Sterols**

  Plant sterols are natural cholesterol like compounds, best known for their ability to lower cholesterol. They are found in plant based foods. It is difficult to get enough plant sterols to achieve any medicinal benefit through a normal diet. Nowadays, many products like juices, margarine and spreads contain added plant sterols. They are designed to replace foods such as butter or margarine that are high in trans fats or saturated fats and cholesterol.

- **Nicotinic Acid/Niacin/Vitamin B**

  The body uses niacin to convert carbohydrates into energy. It helps to boost the health of the digestive system, the nervous system, skin, hair and eyes while increasing the levels of the HDL, or the 'good' cholesterol.

- **Fibre (Psyllium)**

  The seeds and seed husks of the plant Psyllium contain high amounts of fibre and mucilage. Psyllium seeds are used for medicinal purposes. They help to lower the cholesterol and triglyceride levels, prevent or treat atherosclerosis, and support weight loss while helping to prevent or treat obesity. They also help in treating high blood pressure, diabetes, inflammatory bowel syndrome and constipation.

- **Red Yeast Rice**

  Red yeast rice, a substance extracted from rice and fermented with a type of yeast called *Monascus purpureus* has been used as a traditional medicine in China and other Asian countries. It is also used as an additive, food colouring agent and preservative. It contains sterols, Monounsaturated Fatty Acids (MUFAs), isoflavones and ingredients like monacolin-K or lovastatin that help to control cholesterol. The dosage in which it is useful remains unclear and caution is suggested in its use.

- **Green Tea Extract**

  Green tea is tea that has not been fermented. It is said to contain some of the highest amounts of antioxidants out of all the different varieties of tea. Antioxidants decrease the LDL levels in the blood, while raising HDL levels. Green tea slows down the intestinal absorption of cholesterol from the diet, preventing it from entering the bloodstream where it can cause health problems.

- **Policosanol**

  Policosanol, a generic term for the natural extract of plant waxes, is used as a nutritional supplement with the intention of increasing the 'good cholesterol', lowering the 'bad cholesterol' and preventing atherosclerosis.

  However, there is no substitute for a healthy diet. While the jury is out in using Vitamin E in coronary artery disease and beta carotenes have been shown to have marginal effects, foods rich in antioxidants and vitamins like fruits, vegetables and whole grains, have been linked to a reduced risk of heart and blood vessels disease.

- **Chelation Therapy**

  Chelation is a chemical process in which a substance, like a mineral or metal is used to bind to molecules, and adhere to them tightly till they can be ejected from the body.

  The therapy has long been used as a way of ridding the body of toxic metals in cases of mercury and lead poisoning. Its efficacy for the treatment for heart disease remains largely unproven.

The rationale proposed for the use of chelation therapy in heart disease is that the medicine used in the treatment would bind to the calcium in the fatty deposits (plaques) in the arteries. Once the medicine binds to the calcium, the plaques would be swept away as the medicine moves through the bloodstream.

In chelation therapy, a dose of Ethylene Diamine Tetraacetic Acid (EDTA) is administered through an intravenous (IV) line. The medication seeks out and binds to minerals in the bloodstream. The resultant compound leaves the body in the urine.

It must be remembered that the medication used during chelation therapy would bind not just the metals and calcium present in the blood, but also to other minerals that are an important part of the diet. Therefore following chelation therapy, vitamin supplements that contain large amounts of the minerals would be advised to replenish those which the chelation therapy removes from the body. If a person chooses to undergo chelation therapy for heart disease, then it is important that he/she complies with the instructions for taking the vitamins.

No therapy is without inherent risks. The potential side effects of chelation therapy include fever, a burning sensation at the injection site, headache, fall in blood pressure, nausea and vomiting, mineral deficiencies and the inability to create new blood cells. Rarely, permanent kidney damage or failure can occur. In some chelation studies, deaths have also been recorded.

Whether chelation therapy can prevent or treat heart disease remains unclear. Studies are underway but scientific evidence is lacking to support chelation therapy as a treatment for heart disease.

Before opting for chelation therapy as a treatment for heart disease, the risks and benefits (if any) of undergoing the therapy should be carefully considered.

Chapter 7

Make the Right Choices

I. Keep the Heart Happy

Love and the Heart

The body is essentially a chemical factory and love is all about chemistry. Lots of chemicals are released in the brain and body when a person is in love, leading to the feeling that the heart is racing. Believe it or not there is a very real connection between love and the heart. On sighting the one you love the adrenal gland sitting like a cap on the kidneys causes an adrenaline rush. As the hormone flows through the blood the heart beats faster and harder.

Love could actually be dangerous for those with serious heart problems. The increased heart rate and forceful beating increases the oxygen requirement of the heart muscle. In those with plaques, blockages and decreased blood flow the supply demand mismatch can actually precipitate a heart attack.

Dopamine is thought to be the 'pleasure chemical', producing a feeling of bliss. A research team who did brain imaging of people said to be 'madly in love' found activity in the area of the brain that produces the neurotransmitter dopamine.

It has been known for some time that oxytocin or the 'cuddle' or 'love' hormone brings greater heart health. Oxytocin is an endogenous hormone. It is produced by the pituitary gland. The more oxytocin that is released the better is one's ability to handle any stress in life. Oxytocin reduces the amount of stress hormones (primarily cortisol) manufactured by the body. This lowers the blood pressure, which increases in response to anxiety-producing events.

This hormone also seems to reduce the craving for sweets, and drug and alcohol addiction. It is scientifically suggested that oxytocin not only improves heart health but also reduces cell death and inflammation. This helps the heart to heal in case there is any damage.

Another hormone, serotonin that is also secreted, can actually increase the heart rate and blood pressure.

It is then not surprising that the good things in life, like laughter, chocolates, red wine and music have a connection with the heart.

Laughter is the Best Heart Medicine

Research is being carried out as to how laughter protects the heart. What is known is that mental stress causes impairment of the inner lining of the arteries. This results in a series of inflammatory reactions causing fat and cholesterol to build up in the coronary arteries causing a heart attack. Laughter is said to relieve the stress. It helps vascular functioning causing the vessels to dilate, while stress narrows blood vessels.

A study has shown that people with heart disease were 40% less likely to laugh in a variety of situations compared to people of the same age without heart disease.

Chocolate and the Heart

A lot has been said and written about dark chocolate being good for the heart.

Normal bodily processes and contaminants in the environment, like cigarette smoke, form free radicals, which can damage the body cells. To combat the free radicals the body requires antioxidants to control this damage.

Cocoa and chocolate contain flavonols a type of flavonoids, which in addition to having antioxidant capabilities also positively affect vascular health. They can help to lower the blood pressure, make the platelets less sticky and improve the blood flow.

Not just chocolate but other beverages and foods like tea, red wine, apples, cranberries, onions and even peanuts are rich in flavonols.

However, not all forms of chocolate contain high levels of flavanols. Cocoa is processed to produce chocolate. The more it is processed the more flavanols are lost. Most of the commercially available chocolates are highly processed. Chocolate manufacturers are now looking for ways to retain the flavanols.

It was originally suggested that the highest levels of flavaonols were contained in dark chocolate. The fact is that the levels depend on how the dark chocolate is processed, but it is still better to choose dark chocolate over milk chocolate.

It needs to be remembered that chocolates do contain fats and calories. While the calories need to be counted, the fats contained in chocolates are not so bad. However, dark chocolate also needs to be eaten in moderation. Enjoying a piece once in a while need not make one feel guilty.

Other foods rich in flavanols are apples and cranberries.

Red Wine and the Heart

Consuming red wine is said to be good for the heart. The alcohol and antioxidants contained in red wine may be cardio protective. They are said to prevent heart disease by protecting the arteries against damage and increasing the levels of 'good' cholesterol.

The antioxidants like flavonoids or a polyphenol called resveratrol in red wine have been credited with the heart-healthy effects. It is suggested that they prevent damage to the blood vessels, prevent clot formation and decrease the levels of bad cholesterol.

Not just red wine but possibly moderate amounts of other forms of alcohol may also have heart-healthy benefits. It is said to raise the 'good' cholesterol level, reduce clot formation and prevent arterial damage. However more research is needed to support these claims.

However, if you do not drink there is no need to start. Alcohol as a way of preventing heart disease is not advocated.

Alcohol has its own inherent issues. It can be addictive and worsen health problems; the risks of high blood pressure, obesity, liver damage, high triglycerides, certain types of cancer, increase when alcohol is taken in excess. Regular intake of too much alcohol can weaken the heart muscle, causing cardiomyopathy and even heart failure.

If you are already drinking red wine, exercise moderation; for men an average of two drinks a day and for women one drink a day is defined as moderate drinking. A drink being defined as 355 ml of beer, 148 ml of wine or 44 ml of 80-proof distilled spirits.

Music and the Heart

Music therapy for the heart is an idea that is being explored. It has been suggested through various studies that music has an effect on the heart rate and blood pressure. At the end of a hard day soothing music helps one to unwind, relax and de-stress.

An article in 2007 in *The Journal of the American Heart Association*, by Luciano Bernardi, a cardiologist from Italy, suggested that the tempo of the music is the factor that mediates the physiological effect of the music. A fast tempo, whether classical or techno, causes an increase in blood pressure, the heart rate and even the breathing rate, while reducing the baroreflex sensitivity. Slow music, on the other hand, whether classical music or reggae-style, causes the heart rate and the breathing frequency to fall significantly compared to the baseline. Slow-tempo music seemed to lower heart rate more when it followed a faster piece of music than if it came first. Silence between music is said to have the most profound relaxing effect.

It has been suggested that the emotional connect that one may have with the music being listened to can also be important. A musical composition that may be associated with a particularly traumatic event in one's life, even if slow paced could evoke an emotional reaction and actually cause the heart rate, blood pressure and breathing rate to increase.

Companionship

- **Loneliness**

  Man is a social animal, who does not fare well in isolation. Loneliness has detrimental effects on the cardiovascular system. Certain physical changes in the body decrease its ability to fight inflammation, leading to atherosclerosis. In fact research suggests that following certain types of surgery feelings of loneliness dramatically shorten a person's life span.

- **Pets**

  Love does not only come from another human being. Love for pets has also been found to be heart healthy. The social support provided by a pet can make a person feel more relaxed and decrease their stress. Animals may actually improve heart health during stressful situations by lowering blood pressure and regulating the heart rate.

To have a healthy heart and keep the good hormones flowing, one should enjoy life and learn to relax. Enjoy the family, the company of loved ones, laugh, eat healthy chocolate in moderation, drink if you must in moderation and enjoy the music that is life.

II. Prevent and Reverse Heart Disease

Gone are the days when a heart attack meant the end of life, when a heart patient had to be restricted to bed or the house and wait for the inevitable.

Preventing heart disease is in your hands. If you know that you have blockages in the coronary arteries or have already suffered a heart attack take charge of your life and lead a healthier and fuller life.

The mantra for a healthy heart is no different from the mantra for a healthy life.

Albert Einstein has rightly said, "The devil has put a penalty on all things we enjoy in life. Either we suffer in health or we suffer in soul or we get fat."

Moderation and balance are the key.

Eat Healthy, Eat Right

Eat foods low in fat and cholesterol. Saturated and trans fats raise blood cholesterol levels thereby increasing the risk of coronary artery disease.

- A good tip to eating healthy foods is to avoid white foods, i.e., milk and milk products, butter, sugar, *maida* (white flour) and white rice.

- Red meat, palm and coconut oils and dairy products are major sources of saturated fat.

- Bakery products, crackers, margarine and packaged snacks and deep fried foods (*samosas* and *kachoris*) are best avoided. A label that reads, 'Partially Hydrogenated' indicates the presence of trans fats.

- Read the labels when shopping for packaged foods to know the fat and calorie content.

- Choose right. Select foods low in fat and cholesterol. Opt for a diet high in fibre, rich in fruits, vegetables, low fat dairy products and whole grains. Consider eating beans, certain fish and other sources of low-fat protein, nuts and seeds, avocados, olives, rapeseed, sunflower and vegetable oils.

- Cut back on salt. Avoid adding extra salt to the food and do away with the sauces, *papads* and pickles as extras.

Stay Fit, Stay Active

The heart is a muscle. Just like any other muscle it needs to be exercised regularly to stay healthy. Regular exercise tones the heart and body, helps the heart develop more blood flow, keeps cholesterol levels down and helps maintain a healthy blood pressure level.

- For adults, even 30 minutes of brisk walking daily will help reduce the risk.

- Activities such as gardening, using the stairs, housekeeping, even walking the dog all count.

- Children should have 60 minutes of physical activity per day.

- Say no to a sedentary lifestyle. Cut down the time spent watching television.

- Take the stairs instead of the lift, participate or create a physical activity group, walk around the building or exercise during your lunch break.

- It has been shown that even 10 minutes of exercise done thrice a day has the same benefit as a 30 minute continuous work out.

- Encourage schools to serve healthy meals and increase the number of physical education periods in the curriculum.

- Just get up and move. It is important to eat healthy and exercise regularly to maintain a healthy weight. Form support groups of people who exercise together or remind each other to exercise.

Keep a Healthy Weight and a Healthy Shape

Keeping your weight down is important. It reduces the chances of high blood pressure and keeps you active.

Height and weight charts, corrected for age, are available that give the ideal weight for an individual. A calculator can be used to calculate your Body Mass Index (BMI), which tells you whether you are overweight and carry a health risk because of your weight.

Keep the waist to hip ratio < 0.85 in women and < 1 in men to reduce cardiac risk.

Stop Smoking and Avoid Second Hand Smoke

Tobacco and smoking are strictly to be avoided if you want good health. Smoking is a major risk factor for developing atherosclerosis. In persons under the age of 50 it is a major cause of coronary thrombosis.

When you smoke it is a health risk not just to yourself but also to those around you. Even, after the smoker stops smoking, passive smoke stays in the air for several hours.

Second hand smoke is a mixture of two forms of smoke:

- Mainstream smoke which is exhaled by the smoker.
- Side stream smoke comes from the lighted end of a cigarette, pipe or cigar. Side stream smoke contains a higher concentration of cancer-causing agents like nicotine and toxic chemicals. It also has smaller particles compared to mainstream smoke, which make their way into the lungs and the body's cells more easily.

Passive or involuntary smokers are non-smokers who are exposed to this second hand smoke. Non-smokers who breathe in this second hand smoke inhale nicotine and toxic chemicals in the same way as smokers.

Avoid Excess Alcohol

It is important to stay within the recommended guidelines if one consumes alcohol; for men it is three to four units a day and for women two to three units. Binge drinking should be avoided.

Undergo Regular Health Screenings and Check-Ups

A sense of well being or just being lean are not a guarantee of 'no' heart disease. Diabetes, hypertension and abnormal lipid profiles tend to creep up on you. It is important not to adopt an ostrich attitude, 'If I don't know it, I don't have it'. Regular screenings and health check-ups will help early detection and management of any problems to ensure that they are dealt with before any damage is caused.

The following factors should be monitored and controlled:

- **Blood Pressure (BP):** This should be checked at least every two years after the age of 20. If you have pre-hypertension or high blood pressure, your doctor may recommend more frequent screenings, periodic office visits and perhaps regular blood pressure monitoring at home as well. A healthy diet low in saturated fats, regular exercise and taking the prescribed medication regularly should help keep your blood pressure in check.

- **Cholesterol:** A fasting lipoprotein profile (to measure total cholesterol, HDL, LDL and triglycerides) for all adults aged 20 and above, every five years is recommended. Depending on your risk factors for heart disease, your doctor may recommend more frequent testing.

- **Diabetes:** If you have a normal risk for diabetes you should get yourself checked after the age of forty five. If you are aged above 45 years and at risk for type 2 diabetes, you should have your blood sugar checked every year. Also, if you have high blood pressure or high cholesterol, it is important to be tested for diabetes, since diabetes significantly increases your already higher risk of suffering a heart attack. Keeping diabetes under control requires a healthy diet, physical activity, weight control and a regular lifestyle and medication if advised. If you are diabetic, you should monitor your blood pressure closely.

- **Electrocardiogram:** A baseline ECG should be done when you are in your 30s followed by another at the age of 45 to check the health of the heart.
- **Thyroid:** The thyroid gland can cause a number of problems and it is advisable to have the first test at the age of 35 and every five years thereafter for women.

Regular Medication

If you have any underlying medical problems the chances are that you will be taking medication. No matter what is advised or done only a regular, controlled lifestyle and medication will help rein in any problems and ensure a healthy heart.

It is important to take any advised medication regularly. Inform your doctor if you are taking any other medicine, whether allopathic or alternative drugs.

Never discontinue or alter the dosages of any medicine without first consulting the doctor who is treating you.

Stay Happy and Relaxed

Being happy, relaxed and having positive emotions result in biological responses that keep one healthy.

Everybody experiences stress in some form or the other. The difference is in the way the situations are perceived and addressed. We always have a choice in how to react to a situation or emotion. It is important to express oneself yet stay in control. Worrying only gives you stress, it neither changes the situation nor is it the solution.

Stay positive, use positive thoughts to motivate yourself. Setting realistic goals and realizing them is a strong mental booster. Prioritize your tasks so that you do not get pushed into facing deadlines.

Find the ways that help you 'de-stress' best. They could include music, a good movie, an outing with family or friends, going for a long walk, spending time with your pet, and meditation and deep breathing. Do what it takes to laugh, relax and be at peace with yourself.

The *Effect of potentially modifiable risk factors associated with myocardial infarction in 52 countries (the INTERHEART study): case-control study conducted by:* Yusuf S, Hawken S, Ounpuu S, Dans T, Avezum A, Lanas F, McQueen M, Budaj A, Pais P, Varigos J, Lisheng L; published in the Lancet, 2004 Sep 11-17;364(9438):937-52, suggested that abnormal lipids, smoking, hypertension, diabetes, abdominal obesity, psychosocial factors, lack of consumption of fruits, vegetables, and regular alcohol intake alcohol, and lack of regular physical activity account for most of the risk of myocardial infarction worldwide in both sexes and at all ages in all regions. This finding suggests that approaches to prevention can be based on similar principles worldwide and have the potential to prevent most premature cases of myocardial infarction.

III. Live Right

Being healthy and staying healthy is a lot about mind over body. It is important to first be convinced that one should be healthy. This resolve will help one stay on track and not give into temptations. Initially it will often seem that everyone is out to make you forget your resolutions. You decide to control your diet and the office party will be held the next day!

Being healthy becomes a way of life if it is practiced regularly and consciously initially. Thereafter it tends to become second nature. Maintaining a food diary, limiting food portions, allowing 'cheating' occasionally are some ways to start and maintain a healthy regime. Do not procrastinate, start now.

Choose the Right Foods

To stay healthy make the right, informed choices:

- **Consume fewer calories:** Eat moderate amounts of nutrient-rich, low-fat, low-calorie foods. Crash diets, excessive fasting or fancy diets can result in nutritional deficiencies leading to other health problems. Limit the portion sizes.
- **Energy density:** This is the number of calories in a given volume of food. High energy density foods, such as fats,

contain more calories, which means that less volume can be consumed. Low energy density foods can be consumed in bulk as they translate into fewer calories, like most vegetables and some fruits.

- **Make healthy eating a habit:** Vegetables, fruits, grains and lean sources of protein, including beans, fish, low-fat dairy products and lean meats optimize nutrition and taste while promoting a healthy weight.

- **Choose the right carbohydrates:** Make complex, high-fibre carbohydrates, such as whole-grain bread and pasta, brown rice, and other grains, such as oatmeal the source of your carbohydrates.

Avoid
- Products made from white flour, milk and dairy products and white sugar.
- Fast foods, sugary drinks, fatty foods, sweets and desserts.

Increase Physical Activity

An exercise plan to help you lose weight should include regular aerobic exercise, like walking and strength training, such as lifting weights. While structured exercise is ideal a little activity throughout the day will add up and promote a healthy weight.

- Take the stairs - not the elevator.
- Park in the farthest spot in the parking lot.
- Walk or cycle to work or to the store.
- Walk during your lunch hour.
- Play active games instead of watching others play.
- Walk with your family after dinner.
- Do chores manually, e.g., sweep up using a broom rather than a vacuum cleaner.
- Buy an exercise bike and pedal during TV shows or while talking on the phone.
- Use a pedometer and try to increase the number of steps you walk each day.
- Get up and move around. Get up and change the TV channels. Get up and get things do not ask somebody else to get them.

Lifestyle Changes

To lose weight and keep it off needs changes in behaviour patterns.

- One must decide for oneself that weight loss is needed.
- Make lifestyle changes a priority.
- Work to a plan.
- Set small goals.
- Think positive.
- Think and read healthy.
- Avoid food triggers; self-control is the key word.
- Keep a record. A food and activity diary helps reinforce good habits. Important health parameters such as blood pressure, cholesterol levels and overall fitness are of essence, not just losing weight.

Good health is about a life time of maintenance.

IV. Use Technology to Stay Healthy

"Any sufficiently advanced technology is indistinguishable from magic."

— Arthur C. Clarke, *Profiles of the Future: An Inquiry into the Limits of the Possible*

All of us want to be healthy. It is not unusual to start the day, week, month or year with a resolution to maintain a 'healthy lifestyle'. We promise ourselves that we will eat right, exercise right, and have the correct numbers on all our medical tests. This is especially the case if we have just been diagnosed with a health issue like hypertension, diabetes or a thyroid problem or a report has shown up as abnormal.

These good resolutions are often forgotten the moment the first temptation presents itself, like delicious cake, ice cream, sizzling hot *parathas* with butter melting on them, or samosas, to mention a few. The real problem is not when you succumb to the temptation momentarily, the problem stems from not being able to get back on track after the indulgence.

Many people, who are really health conscious and want to stay on top of their health regimes, maintain food diaries, exercise diaries and medication logs. In the past this had to be done manually but today technology has made it easier. With the advent of the mobile phones, computers and other smart electronic devices it is possible to maintain electronic records of your health.

The very act of recording your daily food intake makes you more aware of your eating habits and helps you make better food choices.

Similarly keeping track of how many steps you have walked in a day, the exercise routine that was followed, the number of calories consumed and burnt is an amazing way to monitor your health parameters.

Free calculators allow you to calculate and understand basic health parameters like your BMI, your physiological age vs. your anatomical age (i.e., whether your body tissue is younger or older than your actual age), the waist to hip ratio, to name a few.

Most of these programs are available as free apps on phones or as free downloads on a computer. Ensure that the apps and programs you use are secure so that your medical records are not misused.

Diaries

To keep track of what you are eating, your exercise routine and weight there are diaries available that can be downloaded on a smart phone or computer.

- **Food diaries** can help to calculate your caloric requirements, keep track of the foods consumed and calculate the number of calories in the foods eaten, making you conscious of when you need to balance the calories out.

- **Exercise** diaries help to keep track of the exercise done and calories burnt.

- **Diaries** that keep track of, and represent, your blood pressure and blood sugar levels are also available.

Health Records

- **Personal Health Records (PHRs)** that track all your health parameters are available. It is possible to maintain complete health records from birth through all stages of life. Most such programs available are web-based programs which means, that if required, the information can be shared across geographical barriers. Sitting in India you can get an opinion from a healthcare professional across the globe at a click of the mouse.

Most hospitals today, also maintain **Electronic Medical Records (EMRs)**; this ensures that if you visit the same hospital for all your treatments they can pull up your entire file of all the visits at any time. It also means that any doctor can retrieve your reports at any time if required.

Telecardiology

Many small towns in India do not have a cardiologist. In fact there are only a few thousand cardiologists across the country. Telecardiology enables an individual, or preferably his physician, to consult a cardiologist in another city or town. A lot of individuals come to the bigger cities and towns for their advanced cardiac investigations and procedures and surgeries. On returning home they are managed by their local healthcare professional. A telephone call, fax, email or video that is sent to get an opinion all qualify as telemedicine. At a more advance level, teleconferencing and/or videoconferencing can be arranged to take an opinion or just inform the doctor of the reports. This saves travel time and costs, and allows a number of people to be present at the consultations. Simultaneous, multiple location consultations can also be arranged.

- **Telecardiology Equipment**

  Today there are a number of devices available that have inbuilt transmission capability. How do they work?

  Imagine a blood pressure machine or a glucometer that has bluetooth compatibility and can be linked to your health diaries or health records. If the readings are alarmingly low or high, an SMS or email can be sent to a close relative or even the hospital or treating doctor.

  Home hubs which can be set up at home have an inbuilt capacity to record the ECG, blood pressure, blood sugar, temperature and connect to the health diaries and records where the readings are recorded; they trigger alarms and can even be used for distance monitoring and video-conferencing purposes.

Hand held, tele-ECG machines, the size of a mobile phone, are now available (Fig. 15). They can be used to record a complete ECG. The complete details of the patient are entered and the device can be programmed for various consultants. The ECG is recorded at home, the doctor's clinic or in an ambulance and transmitted to the smart phones of the cardiologists on a free application that can be downloaded (Fig. 16). It is also available as a web based program. The ECG is delivered in less than five minutes of sending it. The cardiologist can report the ECG right from the handset. This ensures an almost immediate evaluation of the ECG by an expert and institution of treatment. Time being imperative if a person suffers a heart attack, definitive treatment needs to be instituted within the golden hour. Worldwide, reports of the use of tele-ECGs have shown significant saving of time and better outcomes in patients suffering heart attacks.

It is important to embrace available technology, wherever possible, to help to keep track of our health. It can help us stay on track, stay motivated, send out alerts in emergencies and get expert advice in the shortest possible time.

Chapter 8

A Personal Account

"Cardiac bypass surgery was the best thing that happened to me. It improved the quality of my life," said Ajit Inamdar, Director and CFO of Cheminova India Ltd.

Inamdar, is a lean, fit, trim 61 year old, who does not look a day over fifty. He was all geared up to run the 2013 'Dream Run' of the Standard Chartered Mumbai Marathon. It sounds very unlikely that he would have needed bypass surgery.

'Work' has been his mantra for as long as he can remember. He enjoys what he does and a loving and supportive family have been his strength.

"Annual medical check-ups are carried out regularly for all employees over the age of 45, so I have been undergoing regular check-ups for the last 15 years. I was diagnosed with mild diabetes in the year 2000, but never had any problems. I took my medications regularly and my blood sugar levels were always well controlled.

During my annual check-up in mid-2009 after my treadmill stress test I was told that there were some borderline changes. I had been following up with my doctor who suggested that we wait before pressing panic buttons.

My father is 90 and has no health issues. My mother underwent a coronary bypass surgery in 1995 and is doing well. I have two siblings. My younger sister was diagnosed with coronary artery disease about a year back and advised an angioplasty. She is on medication now and doing well.

As a part of my follow-up I underwent another treadmill stress test in the beginning of 2010, which also showed some changes. Then in mid 2011, I underwent a stress thallium scan that again showed up changes. Now, I was advised a coronary angiography which I underwent in July 2011. Both the family and I were confident that everything was going to be normal. None of us really took the procedure seriously. I felt fine and had no complaints, but the doctors wanted me to undergo tests. I even felt I was being pushed into unnecessary investigations. Imagine my surprise when I was told that the angiography had shown a blockage in three blood vessels, which could not be treated by an angioplasty. We were all stunned.

It was difficult for me to believe the results. After my third stress test I had travelled to Denmark and Brazil, thirty hour flights, with no problems. The doctors did tell me that it was not an emergency but I needed to get my blocks fixed with surgery. I was still convinced that I was being pushed into unnecessary procedures and couldn't get the thought out of my mind. I wanted a second opinion, even though my cardiologist explained to me that if an angioplasty was possible he would have done it himself and not sent me to another doctor for bypass surgery.

I also decided to look into alternative methods. I read up exhaustively on online articles, explored medicine sites from the US and signed up for an Ayurvedic treatment program. It was a mix of Ayurvedic medicines, exercise, controlled diet and positive thinking to remove the thought from the mind that one had any kind of heart disease. At the treatment centre the CD of my angiography was even played for me and they showed me how the blood continued to flow beyond my blockages. I was told that nature can develop natural new bypass routes and there was no need to worry as the blood flow would automatically be regenerated beyond the blocks.

I was working towards removing the thought that I had blockages in my coronary arteries. There were regular morning walks, yoga and regular eating habits were practiced. In short my lifestyle was undergoing a total change, but after ten days or so I realised I would not be able to live the rest of my life like this. Maybe the therapy was right; every therapy has something going for it.

Now, I was back to square one. I was not confident of the diagnosis. It was almost two weeks since the angiography and I needed to take a decision. I had to get a second opinion, but I didn't know from whom. I received both warranted and unwarranted advice. Everyone I met had a different doctor, a different experience.

Finally, I travelled to Bangalore on the 1st of August to meet a specialist at the Narayan Hrudralay Hospital for a second opinion. The doctor evaluated me and categorically told me that I had only two choices: have a bypass before I have a heart attack or have a bypass after a heart attack. He explained that I was lucky as I had not experienced any signs or symptoms and all my other systems were in excellent condition - but it was time to get a bypass done. That clinched things for me. The moment I stepped out after the consultation, I decided to undergo a coronary bypass at the Asian Heart Institute, Mumbai, and immediately took an appointment.

Being analytical, having some knowledge and being able to understand medical terminology can actually make you indecisive. You need to be convinced before opting for a treatment. However, once the decision was made, there was no looking back. I was mentally prepared. Even the night before the surgery I slept well and was cheerful and smiling even as I went under anesthesia.

The key is to have a positive mind set and be well prepared before the surgery. I had been counselled about the breathing tube and the tubes in my chest that would be necessary after the surgery. I had been taught spirometry breathing exercises prior to the surgery and my physiotherapist had cautioned me saying, 'The spirometer is your friend. Don't forget it post surgery.' I had practiced using it to breathe for two to three days prior to the surgery.

The anesthesiologist had also reassured me when I asked him how I would regain consciousness after the surgery.

I went into surgery with complete faith that nothing would go wrong. I was wheeled in at 8:00 in the morning on 18th August and wheeled out at around 9:30 at night. I did the thumbs up for my family and boss as I was being wheeled from the theatre to the ICCU. I was out of the ICCU on the 20th and home on the 24th.

My family was extremely worried. My wife, both my sons and my daughter-in-law have been pillars of support. They were extremely protective of me post surgery.

I still recall my first baby steps after the surgery. The first time they mobilized me I had my physiotherapist on one side and the ward boy on the other. They actually taught me to walk again.

The physiotherapist came home once a day after the surgery. In fact on the 4th September I climbed three flights of stairs to my parents' house for the Ganpati celebrations with the physiotherapist at my side, and after three weeks of rest, I went to see a movie.

I had also been attending the Brahma Vidya sessions at Vile Parle. The sessions comprised breathing techniques, meditation and the art of positive thinking - a wellness therapy. It is amazing how we start to have so many negative thoughts from a young age. Positive thinking is a must. It is all about mind over body.

In five weeks I was back in the office and even attended the board meeting on the 2nd October.

Three weeks after my surgery, I started my cardiac rehabilitation program. On my first day I heard everyone around me in the cardiac rehab discussing the Mumbai Marathon. Although the 10th Mumbai Marathon was upon us I had always thought that it was not worth it. Since thousands of people ran who would be interested whether anybody else ran or not.

Now after undergoing a bypass, I realised that it was not about what others thought but what I wanted to do. I immediately asked the doctor if I would be able to run. I had six grafts. He told me he would see how I progressed in the next week or so and then decide. I trained for the dream run in the Mumbai Marathon 2013 and was determined to do the half marathon next year.

Today, I work out on the treadmill, cycle, elliptical or do weights thrice a week for one and a half hours. I practice deep breathing for half an hour every morning. Earlier, if you had asked me to do this kind of exercise I would have laughed. I am a workaholic and love what I do. I used to walk for half an hour three or four times a week but that was it. Work was my priority, everything else a waste of time. Today I find the time for exercise and enjoy it. I travel almost twice a week and undertake international travel almost quarterly. Yet, I still exercise wherever I can. My rehab continues and is helping me tremendously.

My diet is much more regulated. We have changed to rice bran oil for cooking. Although there are no restrictions on food, I eat healthy, and if I am hungry I reach out for an extra helping of dal or vegetables rather than an extra roti. The huge gaps between meals have reduced. Although late nights and travel are unavoidable, I get adequate restful sleep, am all charged up and enjoy everything I do. Weekend is family time and we take off to spend time together. I have learned to value what I have more.

Positive thinking, a positive attitude, a healthy lifestyle and being able to control the stress factors are the key to a healthy heart. Of course I still worry about my extended family and friends and still get concerned if they run into problems, but that is part of life.

Finally, I sincerely believe, that having the coronary artery bypass surgery was the best decision I have ever taken."
